have a super l!fe

eat healthy
lose weight
feel great

Talya Lewin

D0494081

Have a Superlife

For information or permission requests, email the publisher or author at haveasuperlife@gmail.com or send your request to Superlife Ltd. Moneyhill Ashbourne, Co. Meath Ireland.

To contact the publisher, visit haveasuperlife@gmail.com.
To contact the author, visit haveasuperlife@gmail.com

Graphic Design: Oded Lavie
Illustration: Nomi Lewin
Cover Design: Studio H

ISBN 978-0-9932403-0-0
Printed in the UK

This book is dedicated to two very special people who are deeply missed in my life

My wonderful father - Abba
Jacques Yossef Lewin
&
My beloved grandmother - Bobbie
Sadie Ratner

Table of Contents

Foreword

by Joshua Rosenthal

We have entered an age where the world is constantly becoming more complex. It is very apparent in the food we eat: we can't pronounce the ingredients on the food we buy, there are thousands of choices in our grocery stores and we are bombarded by advertisements. Food is transported around the globe, and pesticides and chemicals are used to keep food fresher longer and to lengthen its shelf life. All these choices and added ingredients make the simple decision of what to eat overwhelming. The goal of living a healthy, balanced life seems impossible.

Our parents and grandparents lived more simply. They walked into their backyards or community gardens to harvest the food they fed their families. They traded food and goods with neighbors and ate according to the seasons. They cooked meals at home and sat down together for the wholesome family meal.

Many people today are only interested in getting by – eating as cheaply and as quickly as possible. They are living in a "matrix mentality," not questioning what they've been taught, just consuming and adding to the health crisis overtaking the world we live in. One of the most insidious features of this mentality is that life becomes about instant gratification, including the food we eat. The popularity of fast food has grown and so have our waistlines. Obesity is an epidemic. I find it fascinating that people can be so overweight, yet so malnourished. Our world is literally starving for good nutrition.

We all know what is good and healthy for us and what is not. We all are born with that innate intelligence, but everything is stopping us from using it. We set our goals far and our targets too high, expecting instant results, setting ourselves up for failure and frustration.

What Talya Lewin has created in *Have a Superl!fe* is an inspiring, simple, direct approach to living a healthier and happier life. Talya emphasizes that the secret to success is to break down your big goals and aspirations into small, steady baby steps that are absolutely achievable for you, even if it just means drinking one more glass of water a day. She breaks down each step with easy-to-digest information, practical tools that you can use to bring health and vitality back into your life and the lives of your family.

I encourage you to use *Have a Superl!fe* as it is intended, as a compass towards better health, with inspiration and support from the author leading the way.

Joshua Rosenthal, MScEd *is Founder and Director of the Institute for Integrative Nutrition, which teaches the core concepts of Primary Food, Bio-individuality, and over 100 different dietary theories.*

Toward Our Journey

Step by Step
How to Use This Guide

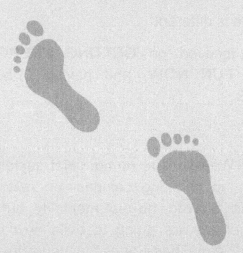

The secret of getting ahead is getting started. The secret of getting started is breaking your complex overwhelming tasks into manageable tasks, and then starting on the first one.

Jim Donovan

In my health counseling practice, I meet many people who have been on and off all kinds of diets for many years – losing weight, gaining it back, losing again only to gain back even more, over and over and over again. People say to me they are like an accordion, stretching and compressing, and left disappointed, frustrated and without hope. Does this sound familiar?

This guide is different!

We are focused on **GETTING ENERGY NOW, HAVING FUN NOW**, and having it be **LONG-LASTING.**

We will have no rigid diet guidelines to follow, no counting calories, no restrictions, no guilt allowed, no diet mentality, but rather together we are going to build new healthy habits, natural basic ones that you actually had as a child and lost somewhere along the way. We will do it just as you learned how to walk: one step at a time, slowly, patiently and with love and support.

This is how it works:

Baby Steps

At the end of each chapter, you choose a **STEP** to take. Do your best to take the step. Make it as big or as small as feels right for you. It is your decision. But I strongly suggest taking **small steps**, breaking down your big step into smaller steps. Then slowly, after you feel comfortable with your initial step, take a bit of a bigger step, and so on. The most important thing is that you are able to actually take the step you choose. I want you to succeed. It is better to succeed with small little steps than fail by choosing too big a step.

Once you succeed you will then be able to move on to a bigger step (or actually, a few small steps together are a big step).

For example: To start, instead of deciding you are going to add a salad to your lunch every day, decide you will add a salad only on Mondays. Once you have established that step, decide you will do it on Mondays and Wednesdays – and succeed at that, too!

Believe me – you will feel great! Then you will be able to do it on Mondays, Wednesdays and Fridays too … and so on. So PLEASE remember: break down your steps.

When **you choose** the step, **be really sure you are able to take that step**. At the very beginning, intentionally break down the step to smaller baby steps.

_ by Step by Step by Step by Step by Step by Step by Step by Step by Step by Step by Step by Step by Step by Step by Step by.....

 ## The Superl!fe Healthy Habit Program Videos That Will Help and Inspire You

I am with you and supporting you not only on paper but on video, too. In 2011 my husband Diarmuid and I opened our Irish-based superfood company "Superl!fe" for unique superfood blends. If you aren't familiar with superfoods, superfoods are extremely potent nutritious foods that can increase your energy levels instantly and transform your health dramatically (i.e. cacao beans, hemp seeds, goji berries and spirulina). We will learn all about them in Step 7.

Throughout the book there are QR codes linking you to great videos that are part of our "Healthy Habit Program", showing you exactly how I make a superfood smoothie, a superfood porridge, basic meals and more. You can access them directly by scanning the code with the camera on your mobile phone.

In some of the videos I use Superl!fe products, but please feel free to use any superfoods of your choice.

Don't fear technology – it is really easy!

All you have to do is download a QR code reader. Here is one option you can try:
http://www.i-nigma.com/Downloadi-nigmaReader .html.

Then use your camera to scan the code, and it will take you directly into the video.

Wow!!! Isn't that amazing?
You can also find our videos at
**youtube.com/user/
haveasuperlife**.

So since we are upgrading everything in our lives, from our car, TV, computer, phones and runners ... why is it that our food is getting worse and worse? Now is the time to upgrade our nutrition, too!

Introduction

*Each man's life represents
the road toward himself.*

Hermann Hesse

The first 34 years of my life were quite difficult. I was born in Israel to a very loving family: a wonderful younger sister, a Belgian father with a great sense of humor and a Canadian mother who made us healthy snacks of cut cucumbers and carrots and is my inspiration for the way I cook and bake. But despite all this, things just always seemed to be hard for me.

As a child I was very shy, clinging to my mother's skirt, and I had no confidence. Throughout primary school, I let my red-haired best friend dominate me and was socially very insecure. I had a horrible fear of standing out, asking the teacher not to ask me anything in front of the class, for fear that I would turn as red as a tomato … which I often did. I was also a poor student.

When I left public school, one of the teachers remarked that I wasn't smart, so in high school, I became obsessed with school and my marks. I was driven to succeed and spent all my days (and nights) studying. Though I was always slim, I became obsessed with my weight and controlled what and how much I ate: drinking Diet Coke, chewing sugar-free gum (waking up in the morning with it stuck to my hair), counting calories, constantly weighing myself, eating low-fat foods and very little in general. I became far too skinny and very low on energy. I also craved sweets.

After graduating from high school, I went swinging

to the other extreme, finding fulfillment in eating two sandwiches in a row, white bread with chocolate spread, chocolate bars, and still chewing lots of gum (eventually my jaw started to click from so much chewing).

Life collapsed when my beloved father suddenly died at the age of 49. I was 18 and a half years old.

Soon after, I found myself in the Far East and fell in love with India. The country of millions of gods, the birthplace of Gautama Buddha felt like home. My encounter with my first Indian guru and spiritual teacher, Osho in Pune, (though Osho left his body two years previous to my arrival) opened a whole new world for me. Meditation, freedom from conforming and, for the first time, learning to be who I am. I started questioning my life – past, future, attachments, choices, God, what I was taught, the ego, my potential, happiness, society, awareness, silence. My life was totally shaken.

For a few years, I became more interested in Being than in Doing. For the first time, I started to go against the flow. While everyone around me was going to university, attaining degrees and getting married, I didn't know what it was I wanted to do. I still had pressure – from outside and within – to go the conventional way. I started studying economics and

Far Eastern studies (and became totally miserable). I looked into Chinese medicine (although studying Chinese medicine and Far Eastern studies in a classroom wasn't for me) and was persuaded to think about law (thank God I didn't even start that). Nothing stuck for very long. I went back and forth to India (about ten times in total) each time finding peace and happiness, then losing it when I got back. Every time I was back home I turned to food for comfort.

At around the age of 24, when I returned to Israel from one of my many trips to India, a friend and I spontaneously opened a cake business together. Since I had always loved baking and always took a cake along with me, it was a very natural thing for me to do. I started the cake business in my mother's kitchen with a carton of apples, a dozen eggs and my mother's apple cake recipe. My friend and I separated as partners, but before I knew it I was baking for all the major coffee shops in Israel. The cake business went really well and supported me through five years of intense film studies and a few different acting schools. I had the business for twelve years.

Although those were years of creativity and inner healing, they were also very demanding, stressful and tough. Running a business, trying to make movies and get a break in the acting world … it wasn't easy, and there were too many disappointments. When I look back on it now, I can see how I was barking up the wrong tree.

For many years I suffered from digestive problems, and one day, while delivering cakes, one of the employees in a coffee shop told me about a Russian couple who healed people through nutrition. I went for a one-hour session … and that was it! The next day I was off coffee, milk products, white flour, white sugar, anything processed and I bought myself a juicer. The healing was extremely quick.

The cake business gave me financial security, but as the years went by and I grew closer to health, I grew further and further away from my cakes. Cottage cheese was switched to tahini, the salads were topped with brown rice and quinoa and as the years went by, I started buying organic produce, becoming very concerned with the way animals were raised and treated. I went on and off being vegetarian.

All that while I was still selling cakes but no longer eating them myself. I also baked healthier cakes, with whole wheat flour, brown sugar and organic eggs, but deep inside I felt that something was very wrong. I wanted to change but didn't have the courage to leave. The cake business became my golden cage.

At 34, my life felt very hard. Between finding myself in long and wrong relationships, painful separations, acting in a play I didn't enjoy (we actually were baking on stage!), trying to make movies and working with the cakes that contradicted my beliefs, something felt fundamentally "out of sync." Although I was doing inner work for many years, I was unfulfilled and unhappy.

Then things changed for me quite instantly and unexpectedly. Though I had been to India so many times, my path never met the path of yoga. One day, while living in a small and noisy apartment in Tel Aviv, I decided to go to a yoga class in a center I had walked by many times, just two minutes away from my home. For some reason, that yoga class was life-transforming. I distinctly remember the feeling after: I felt light and happy for no reason, and that feeling lasted. I remember suddenly realizing that a gray and sad cloud – that I hadn't even been aware of – had disappeared from above my head. Ever since, I have never stopped practicing yoga.

After that day, things began to shift. First, I became

a much happier person and, from somewhere deep inside, decided to remove everything from my life that didn't feel right. Enough of the hard way! I decided to let life show me the way. I decided to go for what happens easily and naturally.

Over the next year, my mother and sister supported the change but all the other people around me thought I was mad. I left the acting, gave up the movies, closed the cake business and went to study nutrition at IIN – the Institute for Integrative Nutrition in New York City. I jumped, and life caught me. I am so grateful. Now life is right. There isn't one thing in my life that feels wrong or compromised.

This book is a collection of everything I have learned over the past 43 years and use in my personal life.

We all have our life "story," but if we have the courage to step out of it, the wisdom not to identify with it so much, the ability to look at it objectively and the incentive to get support, we can create the life we want and deserve.

Though it doesn't happen in one day, it can happen. I honestly now know that life can always be **happier, simpler and healthier**.

While reading this book please:

- **TRUST in LIFE**
- **LISTEN to What LIFE Is Telling You**
- **LISTEN to Your HEART**
- **SLOW Down**
- **Take BABY STEPS**
- **Choose the SIMPLE PATH**
- **BREATHE Deeply**
- **LAUGH**
- **EVERYTHING and ANYTHING Is POSSIBLE**

Let's begin.

Use Your Common Sense

Everyone wants to be healthier, happier, slimmer, more energetic, more focused, more creative. And yet nowadays, even though we are living in such abundance, people are stressed, overworked, eating the worst food, sicker than ever, fatter than ever, depressed, popping all kinds of pills and supplements. We aren't taught how to live a healthy life and what good foods to eat. It is such a pity, since if we use our innate common sense and implement a few simple and practical principles, it is uncomplicated and pretty easy.

New Healthy Habits

My purpose in this book is to give you easy, accessible steps and tools to create new healthy habits in your life and to make changes towards a happier, healthier, more energetic you. We are creatures of habit, for both good and bad. We weren't born brushing our teeth, but we wouldn't dream of waking up and not doing it. In just that same way, you can create new habits in your life, ones that you choose and that will help you live the life you want. At the end of each chapter you will choose one healthy "baby step" to incorporate into your life. Eventually each may become a habit. In the beginning, resistance might arise. At first it could be quite strong, but it may actually be a sign that you are on the right path. If you are ready for it, you could try to observe that resistance, letting it be, instead of reacting.

A tip for dealing with resistance: The smaller the steps you take, the less the resistance.

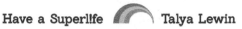

This Is Not a Diet - Diets Don't Work!

For me today, it is so simple, fun, tasty and quick to eat healthily, but many people don't seem to have the tools, knowledge or stamina to go for it. Others have their own fixed ideas of what it means: "hard work," "you are not allowed foods you love," "not tasty," "diet mentality," "expensive" and so on. Actually, it is totally the contrary. Eating in a healthy way is the easiest, tastiest, cheapest and most sustainable way to live today. And it certainly isn't a diet.

During my high school years, I was constantly on a diet: counting calories, drinking Diet Coke, eating very little, feeling low on energy, unhappy, craving sweets and constantly thinking about food. In the long run, **diets don't work!** They operate like a pendulum – you swing to one extreme and then find yourself soon after swinging to the other extreme. There are also so many different diets, each one emphasizing that their way is the only and right way. In my life I integrate everything and don't have any one way. What I am talking about is a lifestyle, one that will make you feel and look so great that it will be obvious to you that you are on the right track.

Adding

Our focus will be on what we are adding, not on what we want to subtract.

For example: Instead of focusing on drinking less coffee, we will focus on eating and drinking foods that will give you so much energy that you will not need the coffee. Instead of focusing on eating less chocolate, (I love chocolate, and we will add healthy chocolate) we will add foods that will be sweet, delicious and healthy – you will not need the sugary chocolate bar. We will substitute unhealthy food with the healthy version. You will learn to ask yourself: What healthier option can I eat?

Focusing on the HOW

There are many good books on the market about health and nutrition, but we are going to focus on **HOW** to eat and live healthy. The **WHYs**, though they are important, are not our emphases here. If you picked up this book, you likely already know why it is important to put good food into this amazing body of yours and you have the desire to do so. However, if you still want more information, please refer to my list of recommended books on page 299.

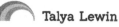

Make It Yours

Healthy eating can become just as simple and user-friendly as eating junk and instant foods. In my nutrition counseling practice, I have seen that when I show people the path that works for me, it often works wonders for them. So if you are ready to upgrade your life and nutrition, you're in luck, because I am going to take your hand and walk you through HOW I do it, step by step. I will give you a push in the right direction, a little information, hopefully a lot of inspiration, and the tools you require to continue.

But I want to emphasize that we are all different, and there isn't only one right way of eating. It's not important to do it exactly my way but rather to take the tools and use them in ways that work best for you. Take what resonates, switch things around, add your own variations and ditch the rest. It must feel right. **It must work for you** and suit your lifestyle, your body and your own likes and dislikes. Our focus is on making this sustainable, a lifelong way of eating and living.

Be Patient With Yourself

Remember that you will be learning a new language and, like any new thing, it takes practice, persistence, patience and flexibility. You have been living a certain way for many years. Deep changes take time, especially when we are introducing new dietary and lifestyle habits. As the saying goes, *"Rome wasn't built in a day."*

The good news is that it is totally possible to change, as long as we don't look for instant results and gratification and we know that it is a process. If you happen to take a few wrong turns or "fall off the wagon," try not to judge yourself too harshly. It is all part of the journey. It is neither good nor bad – it just is what it is. It is very important to always be gentle and loving to yourself and focus on what you are achieving. Instead of being upset about what isn't going well, ask, *What is going well? What have I accomplished so far?*

It Is About Progress, Not Perfection

My mentor and teacher, Joshua Rosenthal, the founder and director of the Institute for Integrative Nutrition in New York City, always says, ***"It isn't about perfection. It is about progress."*** I used to try and perfect everything I did, and it destroyed all the pleasure. I suggest taking baby steps, making small changes and focusing on your progress. Forget about perfection. After a while you will suddenly be surprised and excited to see that you are on a different YOU planet.

Slow Down

In our fast-paced world, we all want everything to be instant (instant coffee, microwaved food, fast foods, instant reality celebrities). We do everything fast and look for quick results. I still remind myself to "hold my horses". As the saying goes, *"haste is of the devil."* I want to invite you to look at this as a lifelong journey, to let the change be gradual. Even if you read the book in one go, take the steps slowly. Don't try to implement everything all at once. Take one thing at a time, bring it into your life, master it, feel comfortable with the new habit and then add another.

Research shows that it can take 21-60 days to create a new habit. Even if you add only one new healthy habit a month, if you reread this book several times over the course of a few months, creating new habits with each reading – you are doing great! When we make changes or add new habits, resistance can arise. With time, it will lessen, and the practice will actually become easy.

Awareness

On this journey, together we will slowly learn how to bring the awareness back to what we eat, how we eat, how we feel and how we live. When we slow down, we may gain back the connection to our food, our bodies, our instincts, our planet, our lives.

Take Fun Baby Steps – in the NOW!

Life is all about the steps we take **now**. We must have fun and enjoy the process of getting wherever we are heading, because **if it isn't fun, it isn't healthy** and **it won't last**. I always remind myself, *The steps of getting there are the qualities of being there.* This is a bit hard to understand but is an important hidden secret: how you feel along the way actually determines how you will feel once you arrive. That means that you must enjoy the way or the steps, and then you will also enjoy the destination once you get there. If you don't enjoy the process along the way, then you won't enjoy it once you get there either, and then it won't last. Though you may reach your goal, all will vanish a few months down the road if it wasn't attained through a joyful process. *We have all been there, we have all done that* … haven't we? That is why dieting doesn't work, pursued under a stressful, rigid mentality. So please, having your goal in mind, put all the emphasis on the NOW, on the steps, on it being exciting, fun and easy for you, so it can manifest naturally and last your lifetime.

Simplicity is King

I believe in choosing the simple path, the one of least resistance. It doesn't mean doing nothing;

it means not complicating things, keeping things simple. Many times when we want to achieve something, we will jump head over heels to get it, sometimes really complicating things – I used to do that. Nowadays I feel that nothing complicated is worth my while. Usually there is an easy and simple path we can choose. Always ask yourself, *How can I simplify this? How can I break it down to smaller steps? How can I make it easy, fun and enjoyable for me?*

You Are the Focus

Place the focus on yourself, on what feels good and right for you, and less on satisfying the people with whom you come into contact – your family, friends, co-workers and so on. It doesn't mean you become negatively egoistic or self-centered, but rather, without hurting anyone else, you do what is right for you. You listen to your inner voice, your instincts, your desires, likes and dislikes. Many of us (and I have been there, too) try to please people. But often, we pay a price for that. And in the long run those people pay a price too. The beauty is that when you do what is good and right for you, it usually is good for everyone else.

Calmness

Last but not least. Often, when people start changing their habits, especially when it is connected to food, rigidness and stress take over. You start saying to yourself, *No more coffee! This is my last piece of cake, my last pizza. From now on only water and vegetables. I will go to the gym every day...* And there goes all the pleasure in life, and stress takes over.

I want to emphasize: *Let things happen on their own!* **Continue eating and living exactly as you are** and walk the path we will be taking together. Often the thing itself may be easy, but it is the thoughts and rigid decisions that make it harder than what it really is. For example: Have your coffee, but have it later in the day (having coffee first thing in the morning on an empty stomach is very unhealthy). Remind yourself that everything is okay as it is. All you have to do is breathe, be opened-minded, be calm and take gradual little steps that suit you. Then you can commit to slowly adding different foods and habits into your life. Let the rest happen on its own.

Excited?! Are You Ready?

- Are you ready to live a life with more energy?
- With a higher level of happiness?
- More excitement?
- More focus?
- Greater health?
- In a body that feels comfortable?
- Are you ready to live the life of your dreams?

If you are ready to make a change, write 'Yes!'

_____

Congratulations!!! You just took your first step.

Please trust me, and I promise you, you will upgrade your life.

With health, love and inspiration,

Talya Lewin

> I recommend using this book like a notebook: write in it, scribble, make notes and mark things that are important to you.

Step

2

Standing Up To Your Word

Use the power of your word in the direction of truth and love.

The Four Agreements

This is one of the strongest, most important steps of all. And that is why it is the second step we will take. Words have power. What we say actually has energy and can manifest. If we start noticing what we say, say only things we will actually do and then do what we say we will do – just that on its own can be life-transforming. It is amazing to be that kind of person, and it actually mostly benefits you.

I am sure you are familiar with people who really do whatever they say they will do. And then there are others you know who don't. You have to ask them if they did it, check up on them, remind them or sometimes you just let it all go from the start. You don't take what they say seriously.

> How would you feel and what would your life look like if you were to always stand up to what you said you would do, big or small, whether it is to yourself or to other people? Stand up to your word. Wouldn't that be one great healthy habit!

For many years I have had integrity with my word. I always do what I say I will do – it gives me so much satisfaction, power, inner strength and energy. People know they can trust me, and mostly I know I can trust myself. I will not commit to something I know I can't or don't want to do. I will just say no. It is better to say no than to say you will and then not do it.

For this reason, I recommend that on this journey we are taking together, break down the steps you will commit to into small, possible, baby steps that you really can do. And do them! As suggested in the previous chapter, make them even smaller than what you originally think you can do. For example: instead of deciding you will walk every day for one hour, decide you will walk at first for 15 minutes, maybe twice a week. You can always walk more, if it works out but master that and then commit to more.

So, your second and most important step is **having integrity with your word**.

Pay close attention to what you say, and commit to and do what you say you will do, whether it is for your family, friends, colleagues or yourself.

Step
2

Please sign this personal contract with yourself.

I commit that I will pay close attention to what I say and what I commit to, whether it is for myself or my family, friends or colleagues. I will do my best to stand up to my word.

Please sign here: _____

Staying In The Positive Zone

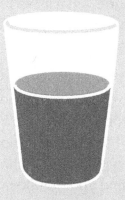

*If you can find a path with no obstacles,
it probably doesn't lead anywhere.*

Frank A. Clark

In my early twenties, a friend gave me a cassette that someone had recorded. (Yup! Not so long ago we were still using cassettes!) On it was handwritten, "Positive Thinking." I listened to it while driving in my car. Since I was quite young, I was very open and fresh to these new ideas. It was all about the difference between people who are happy and successful and people who aren't, what we focus on, and the language we use with ourselves on a daily basis (positive or negative talk). At the time it was very interesting to me, but I think it took many more years and hardships to be able to implement it.

Don't we all have that inner conversation that pulls us down and takes us to "places" we have visited so many times but aren't good for us? How many times have you found yourself in front of the open fridge, gazing in – eating standing up, eating unhealthy foods, eating in a rush – just to find yourself 30 minutes later feeling stuffed and guilty? Going to food is the easiest way to escape, and we all do it (or have done it at some time in our life). But how would you feel if you didn't go to food when you felt stressed, alone, disappointed, angry, guilty, tired or low?

Whether connected to food or not, getting yourself out of the "hole" once you fall in isn't easy. To keep myself in the positive zone and really help myself succeed and be happy, I have a few tools that I have been using over the years. These tools slowly transform the mind so that eventually it will go to the positive automatically.

The first step is to **be aware of those other voices**, the ones in your head that you have been listening to for years. You trust and believe in them, but they aren't getting you anywhere. On the contrary, they drag you down; they are pessimistic, exaggerated, untrue voices. (They say things like, "You are ugly," "You are a loser," "You can't do this," "You aren't smart enough," "You never succeed," "You are a bad person," "You are fat," "You will never make it.")

The second step is telling those voices in your head, **"Thank you for sharing, but …,"** **"Come back tomorrow,"** **"Come back later,"** **"I am busy now."** The main thing is not to put too much emphasis on fighting the voices that are pulling you down, but rather thank them for sharing and move on. The more you listen to them and believe them, the stronger they will become. The more you fight them, the more powerful they will become. Giving them attention will make them lose their strength and eventually dissolve. Often, it is enough to be aware of the voices to make them slowly vanish. Think of it like a fire. Fighting or listening to those voices is like throwing wood into a fire – the more wood you add, the stronger and hotter the fire will become. But if you just watch the fire, without throwing in any more wood, slowly the fire will burn itself out.

The third and important step is bringing in **optimistic uplifting thoughts or affirmations** that will get you out of the rut and pull positive energy and your wants into your life. It is so much easier to live life being optimistic and joyful. The important thing is not only to say these affirmations in your mind and thoughts but to really bring them into your whole body, to feel them throughout. Otherwise it will just be an intellectual exercise, and they won't have the impact you want. With this step I follow a few different ways to help me stay happy, motivated and inspired:

1. **Focus on the positive in your life.** There are always positive things happening to us, but we often forget to notice them, take them for granted, dismiss them or belittle them. Whatever we focus on grows, exactly like watering a plant. If we focus on the "negative" things in our life, the things that pull us down, that is what we are watering and that is exactly what will grow. On the other hand, if we focus on the positive things, remind ourselves what is good in our life, what we are lucky and grateful for – and not just say it but sincerely feel

it – that is exactly what we will get more of. We are like magnets: We attract what we focus on. So, pull into your life whatever you want more of.

2. **Make an uplifting chart*.** This is a very helpful tool that I have used for a long time. It programs your mind to shift from the negative way of thinking to the positive. For years my mind was very negative. So often I saw the half-empty cup. It was already an automatic response. It was my default option. The first step for me was noticing the pessimistic thoughts and how they were totally shaping, creating and controlling my life and suppressing my happiness. The second step was changing them to positive, true, reasonable thoughts. Here is the easiest way I found to do it. Every time you notice a negative thought, wherever you are, take a piece of paper (use your notebook, diary or even a napkin) and draw a line down the middle. Write Negative, Destructive Thoughts at the top of the first column and Positive, Constructive Thoughts at the top of the second. In the first column write down your negative thoughts. Do it without thinking – just let your thoughts flow onto the paper. No one is going to read it. You will throw it out afterwards.

---

* Inspired from the book "Feeling Good" by David D. Burns.

These thoughts are usually pessimistic, unrealistic, exaggerated, unreasonable lies. Yes, **LIES**!! They aren't true, but we believe them. The first column could be something like, *I am fat and ugly. I am a loser. I am stupid. I will never succeed at anything I do. I am old. I will always be alone. I will never find/do/be … I have no friends. No one likes me …* After pouring out all the negative thoughts that are at that moment in your mind, read them over and ask yourself if they are really true. You might notice that some have truths but are really exaggerated. Then go to the second column and write down contradictory, positive, realistic, reasonable truths. Yes, only truths!

The second column could be something like, *I am not fat; maybe I could lose a few pounds, but I am far from being fat and I'm certainly not ugly. I actually have beautiful eyes and great skin. I'm not a loser. I might be having a hard time now, but eventually things will work out. I am really succeeding now at … And X/Y/Z is actually going really well.*

The more you do this, the more your brain will get used to thinking in a positive manner and eventually you won't have to fill in the chart anymore, or you will do it in your head without a pen and paper.

However, to begin with, I strongly recommend just taking a piece of paper and a pen and writing – it is that easy! Don't listen to the thoughts in your head that may be trying to convince you otherwise (thoughts like, *What is the point? This is stupid. It might be good but not for me. I'll do it later*).

Just do it! Try it a few times and notice if your mood shifts after writing down the positive part. Notice how you feel after writing down the Negative, Destructive Thoughts versus how you feel after writing down the Positive, Constructive Thoughts. You will have to do it for a while, until it gradually becomes your brain's new default option of thinking.

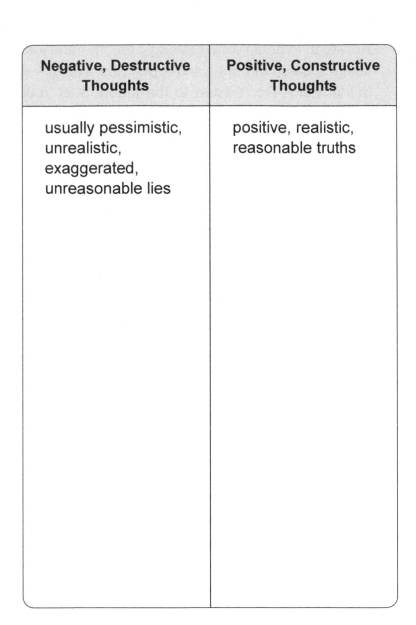

Negative, Destructive Thoughts	Positive, Constructive Thoughts
usually pessimistic, unrealistic, exaggerated, unreasonable lies	positive, realistic, reasonable truths

3. **Feel your body's sensations and emotions.** I don't imply that we should fight or dismiss our thoughts and feelings; however, sometimes we see life through pessimistic glasses, and it is helpful to clean them a bit or actually change them to optimistic ones. Yet it is also very important to give space to our true feelings and emotions, to feel what it is we are going through right NOW. Once we let ourselves really feel our deep emotions and physical sensations, they often resolve themselves (even though at first they might intensify). From my experience, it is beneficial to put our thoughts aside and focus on the feeling and emotion (sadness, anger, jealousy, fear) and the body's sensations. Thoughts and feelings manifest in the body as physical sensations (backache, stiff neck, tension, pain, sweat, warmth, chills, tingling, pressure). Without doing anything, just let yourself observe the feelings and sensations of your body, without the thoughts. Let yourself really feel what is happening. Don't fight it. It can be helpful to close your eyes and observe. Often, after deeply focusing on what you are feeling and on your body sensations, they will pass like a wave, and a greater happiness will arise.

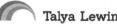

4. **Use quotes.** Use other people's quotes or your own sayings. Really feel them. It isn't enough just to say them automatically – the trick is to bring them into your body, to say and feel them emotionally. That is the way! I have some inspiring quotes hanging above my computer, like, *"Anything is possible."* How inspiring and exciting is it to feel THAT 20 times a day? The great thing is that the more you intentionally use them, the more they become a part of you and the less you will need them. They become new voices in your head and eventually become automatic, pushing aside the old destructive voices. To help remind yourself in the beginning, I advise writing out and hanging them up in visible places: near your computer, on the fridge, on the mirror, in your diary, on the dashboard of the car or anywhere else that helps you see and use them when needed. Try using the ones below or make up your own.

"It isn't about perfection. It is about progress."
Joshua Rosenthal

"The steps of getting there are the qualities of being there."
Anonymous

People don't always get this amazing saying. Just

to remind you again, since I use this one often: The way we behave in the steps towards getting anything represent the qualities we will have once we arrive. So if you are stressed, nervous and unhappy while you are on your way towards wherever you are heading, those are the qualities you will have once you get there. But if you are calm, happy and enjoying the way, then those are the qualities you will have when you reach your goal.

"In the broad picture of my life, how important really is this?"

We identify so strongly with our life that it is very helpful to zoom out and ask ourselves that question. It gives perspective. And often, what seems so horrible at that moment isn't such a big deal in the long run and in the broad picture. In many cases, it was actually the best thing that could have happened. It had a purpose.

"Anything is possible ..."

So inspiring and so true. We really can achieve anything we put our minds to – slowly, patiently, persistently and with trust, even if there are challenges and detours along the way.

"Don't take anything personally."

Nothing really is personal. Each person is living his or her own life with his or her own story. Many times, the way people behave towards us has nothing to do with us, even if it is directed towards us.

"Don't cry because it is over; smile because it happened."

Good things always do come by again. We tend to forget that. We forget that life is constantly changing. Nothing stays as it is. Like a field that has weeds or flowers growing in it, if you pull them out, something new will always grow there. The field will never stay bare. It always helps to be grateful for what we had, even if it is over. Gratitude for anything brings more of what we are grateful for. Instead of focusing on what is over, we can remind ourselves that things are changing all the time and be excited about the new, unknown good thing that will be growing in the field and coming our way.

"I'm bringing the power back to me."

Put the focus on **YOU**. Bring the power back to you. Often when something doesn't happen the way we want, if we reflect on it with honesty, we will see and admit that it isn't what we truly wanted.

Then we gain back our power and are freed from being the victim.

"I walk my talk."

It is so strengthening to be and do what we believe and preach. That is why I had to leave my cake business. It wasn't in accordance with "My Talk." Believe me, there is nothing better than living a life that is totally "Your Talk."

Add some of your own strong truths:

1.

2.

3.

4.

5.

Which of the options in Step 3 are you choosing in order to keep yourself in a positive half-full cup mode?

Instead of turning to food, how will you focus on the good in your life?

Will you make an uplifting chart?

Will you feel your body's sensations and emotions? Will you use quotes?

What can you do to make your life be more like "Your Talk"?

Basic Health Information
Your ABC

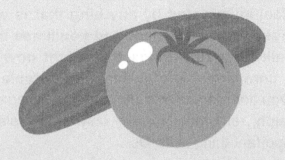

To eat is a necessity,
but to eat intelligently is an art.

Francois de La Rochefoucauld

You thought you had bought a guide that deals with food … well, you did, and at last we are at a chapter about nutrition. While this guide is more about **HOW** to eat and be healthy and less about **WHY**, like cement that holds building blocks together, good information helps us make the right choices and stick to them. So here is some basic WHY knowledge that I hope will help you upgrade to healthier living.

Before we go on, I would like to emphasize the very important note at the end of the chapter: **Please don't feel intimidated by anything that is written here. Take what feels right and you'll see that as you walk the path, things that might now seem totally unreasonable may feel comfortable later**. While you are reading this chapter, if anything seems **Too Much**, remember to take only what feels right. The important thing is **To Do**.

Nutrition is one of the weirdest sciences out there. It is the only science where research can come out with scientifically proven contradicting results every other day – and seemingly every one is right. No wonder we all are so confused. However, when it comes to health information, don't trust just anyone, certainly not the big food companies who frankly care more about making money than about our health. I strongly recommend researching information, educating yourself, reading labels, waking up and questioning the "fuel" you put into your body, our vehicle for this life's journey. Would you ever put the wrong gas in your car?

> **Food for Thought**: We actually are different than our cars. Every part of our body – our bones, skin, hair, brain, cells, everything! – is constantly renewing itself, all the time, mostly from the food we eat.

THE *NOS* TO KNOW

Microwave (go back to a stove)

There has been enough research proving that microwave ovens aren't as innocent as we think: They distort the molecular structure of foods, cause food to be toxic and carcinogenic, destroy most of the nutrients and create many other health problems. Would you still use a microwave if it were called a radiation oven? There is no gentle way to put this: Throw the microwave out!! Or wrap it up with a ribbon and give it to someone you don't like at all, though personally I wouldn't even give it to my enemy. Instead of the instant micro-zap, re-warm, steam or cook your food like in the good old days: in a covered pot with a little water, on the stovetop.

💡 Tip:

With leftovers, forget the plastic containers – just put them back in the pot and, once cooled, place the pot in the fridge to use later; this saves on both energy and your washing-up time.

> **Food for Thought:** A stove will take up a few more minutes of your life but it might lengthen your life by many minutes.

Plastic containers (switch-up to glass)

Molecules of the chemicals in plastics may leech into foods and beverages. This transfer especially occurs with oils, which "melt" the plastic, or when re-heating. I recommend storing your food in glass jars (then you can also see what's inside) and always buying food, especially oils, nut pastes and acidic foods, in glass containers. Other good storage options are ceramic, porcelain or stainless steel. Bought water is better when in a glass bottle, or if you have a home water filter, you can carry around a refillable stainless steel bottle.

Sugar and artificial sweeteners (switch-up to raw honey, grade B maple syrup, silan date honey, date sugar, xylitol, real stevia or organic cane sugar)

White processed sugar is something to stay away from. It is called "the white thief" or "empty calories" (since it has only calories, no nutrients whatsoever) and is actually very addictive. No wonder all the major food companies intentionally put lots of sugar in their products (from chocolate and sweets through to bread, ketchup, pasta and even in toothpaste). Sugar raises our insulin level instantly; overconsumption is directly linked to type 2 diabetes and other diseases. Its long list of side effects includes suppressing the immune system, interfering with absorption of minerals, depression, obesity and much more. Artificial sweeteners are even worse. They can cause cancer and are loaded with well-recognized neurotoxins. Their symptoms can be headaches, memory loss and eye problems, just to name a few. They also increase your appetite, making you eat much more than you really need. People who eat diet foods (food sweetened with artificial sweeteners) find themselves with uncontrollable eating attacks. Our body is created to **eat whole foods**, foods that are as nature created, **not "diet" foods**. When we eat whole foods, we feel satisfied, but when we eat diet foods (foods that are so empty and unnatural), our bodies cry for nutrients. And then often we can't stop eating. So enjoy switching up to natural sweeteners, but remember that all sweeteners should be used in moderation.

> **Food for Thought:** Have you ever seen a person eat just one diet cookie? A bit of diet cheese? How many people do you know who eat diet foods and drink diet sodas are really slim, happy and healthy?

Sodas and diet drinks (switch-up to water)

This is one big NO!! Here, there is no question. Do not get close to this junk. Soda drinks are made from carbonated water (plain water infused with carbon dioxide, creating artificial bubbles), caramel coloring, synthetic caffeine (worse than the natural stuff), phosphoric acid and taste enhancers and loaded with high-fructose corn syrup and sugar. One can of soda can have up to 10 teaspoons of sugar. Sugar actually dehydrates the body, making you crave more liquid and drink more pop, until YOU pop. Switch to water and, if you don't like the pure taste, add some mint leaves, a slice of cucumber, chia seeds, real lemon or a little natural juice (not the preserved stuff).

 Tip:

In the morning, 30 minutes before breakfast, drink one glass of lukewarm water with freshly squeezed lemon juice.

Processed foods (switch-up to natural whole foods)

In the last 60 years, our food has changed dramatically, but the biology of our bodies has stayed the same since man walked the earth. Our bodies are designed to eat real foods that nature and the earth created: full of fiber, minerals, vitamins and antioxidants. The endless shelves of foods that you find in supermarkets today are very far from what your great-grandmother ate. They are processed, stripped of all the fiber and most of their nutrients, heated, preserved, concentrated, fortified with lab-created vitamins and minerals and seemingly able to sit for months on the shelf without going bad. They are loaded with sugar, salt, rancid oils, food coloring, taste enhancers, MSG, preservatives, and the list goes on. I call those foods *dead food*. They look like food, some of them might taste like food, but they don't have any life energy in them. I recommend buying foods that have a shorter shelf life but have life in them and will lengthen your life, foods that have enzymes (life force) and will actually go bad after a few days. Add more natural whole foods (vegetables, fruits, nuts, seeds, whole grains, legumes) and stay away from all the processed, preserved, boxed, canned, bottled, dead poison.

Food for Thought: If food has no life energy in it and can sit for months on the shelf and not go bad, what do you actually get from eating it?

Hydrogenated low quality vegetable oils (switch-up to healthy oils)

We are all brainwashed to believe that oil is "bad" for us and that everything should be low-fat, oil-free. Well, here is the secret: It all depends on the kind of oil you consume. Good oils are good for you, while the bad ones stick to your hips and clog your arteries. Don't believe the advertisements on TV about healthy margarine (you might be better off eating plastic). Stay away from **processed,** hydrogenated, trans-fats and **oils that are used in industrialized, packaged foods, the cheap, low-quality oils: soybean, corn, sunflower, canola and other vegetable oils and margarine. They are extremely damaging** to the body. Though symptoms may not be felt, results can include cell damage, premature aging and many other problems.

The healthy oils – olive, coconut and fats from whole foods like avocado, seeds, nuts, nut butters, coconuts and olives – are important for vitamin absorption and metabolism. They assist our body by helping to stabilize our weight and nourish our skin, hair and nails. I recommend using certified organic, cold-pressed, extra-virgin and unrefined oils. Look for dark glass bottles (since light, heat and air oxidizes oils), and store in a cool, dark place (not near the stove or in the sun). **Don't fear oil.**

Food for Thought: You would never put the wrong oil in your car, but the right one is essential!

Processed table salt (switch-up to pink Himalayan or sea salt)

All salt originates in the sea, and natural sea salt contains up to 60 important trace minerals. Most people use common table salt, which has been refined and stripped of many of these minerals and is really harmful for the body, causing many side effects, accumulating liquids in the tissues, joints and kidneys, raising blood pressure, drying out the body and contributing to weight gain.

Do your body and yourself a favor. Throw out your harmful, chlorine-bleached table salt, which contains mostly sodium chloride and manmade chemicals (like moisture absorbents) and go get yourself some sea salt or Himalayan salt (one of the healthiest salts). Both have many beneficial trace minerals. Healthy salt has a pink or grey shade, so look for color.

 Tip:

There is a lot of refined salt used in restaurants and packaged foods. You can't control the amount of salt when you eat out but you certainly can control both the amount and quality that you put in your homemade food.

Read Labels - Be a Food Detective

One of the important steps in taking control of our health is reading the labels of the food we buy. Even if the label says *Organic, Natural, Healthy,* always read the ingredient list. When you do buy organic, make sure it has a stamp of the organization controlling organic produce in your country. Reading labels isn't as easy as it may seem, and many of the ingredients can be written in a misleading way.

Here are a few detective tips:

- Whatever is listed first is the main ingredient. You will be shocked to learn that most of the processed foods have sugar (under its many different names), salt and oils (vegetable oil can mean margarine and other unhealthy oils) listed in the first four ingredients. Stay away from foods that have an ingredient list that is very long and includes all kinds of names you don't even know how to pronounce and all kinds of letters with numbers, like E202, E339 …

- Invisible toxic chemical words you would like to stay away from are MSG, flavorings/ colorings (even if written "natural" doesn't mean it is healthy), sodium nitrate (a white crystalline salt – used in the manufacture of gunpowder, explosives, fertilizers and for curing meats).

- Take one of your packaged foods and Google each ingredient. You might be surprised to find out what is actually in your food.

Sorry about all the *no*s – let's now go to some of the *yes*es…

THE *YES*ES TO YES

Switch-up to organic

Do you think it is crazy to eat organic? Well, I actually think it is crazy not to. Why would you want to eat food grown with synthetic pesticides, herbicides, fungicides, petroleum-based fertilizers, chemicals, antibiotics, hormones, genetically-modified genes and traces of heavy metals? Or food that has been irradiated? Not so long ago all foods were "organic." Nowadays, all the "conventional" food (from both the vegetable and animal kingdom) is full of pollutants and toxins, causing cancer and diseases of the thyroid, liver, kidney and blood, burdening the immune system.

When I tell people I eat organic, many times the response is that it isn't 100 percent organic and that I'm crazy to spend all that money. Well, if it took us sixty years to destroy our food, it is going to take some time to heal, but it will only happen when more people say NO to foods grown with all those toxins and make intelligent choices towards natural, organically grown and humanely raised foods.

I don't think I'm the crazy one. If those toxins kill all kinds of insects, weeds and pests, what does it do to us and to our kids over a lifetime, and to the entire food chain of the planet?

 Food for Thought: Would you spray your salad with a spray against cockroaches? Isn't it kind of the same thing?

Tip:

When buying organic, try and find a co-op in your area, an organic market or an organic farmer who brings the food straight to your house. When buying in a store, make sure it has the organic stamp or seal of the organization that controls organic produce in your country. I love receiving my weekly organic box straight from the farmer. It arrives freshly picked, still has sand on it and even caterpillars here and there. When I see a live caterpillar or bug walking on the green leaves, it is always a good sign. If it comes to a choice, I'd personally rather spend my money on good food and have fewer shoes and drive an older car...

Switch-up to humanely raised and organic products from the Animal Kingdom

In our world today, we have turned animals into machines. It is easy to shut our eyes to that reality since, for most people, animal products taste really good. But it is time to wake up, take off our shades and look the truth straight in the eye. In today's world, cows are no more than milk, cheese and hamburger machines. Chickens are egg, schnitzel and roasted chicken machines. They live in horrible, miserable conditions (focusing on that reality is what helps me reduce my consumption of most animal products), are pumped with antibiotics and hormones and are fed food that isn't right for them, making them sicker. Even if you don't want to be a vegetarian, what kind of energy do you think is in an egg laid by a chicken that lives in total suffering and pain, pumped with antibiotics? What is actually in that white liquid we call milk when it is produced by an enslaved, sick cow, loaded with hormones and antibiotics?

Ask yourself what stands behind the product. Don't be fooled by big corporations who are selling a beautiful image, through manipulative advertising, smart marketing and colorful packaging, of happy cows grazing green fields or of fluffy white hens. The reality is very far from that. It actually is the total opposite. But if those real pictures WERE on the package and in their advertising, who would buy them? Consider caring about how the animal is raised and remember: whatever the animal absorbed in its lifetime, we absorb in turn when we eat it. There are many healthy, vegetarian, animal-friendly, vegetable protein options. If you do choose to eat animal products, I would strongly suggest to reduce the amounts and choose those that are organic and humanely raised!

If slaughterhouses had windows, everyone would be vegetarian!

Hesh Goldstein

To really get what is happening in the animal food world, watch this lecture on YouTube:

Best Speech You Will Ever Hear – Garry Yorovsky

Switch to healthy cleaning products

We aren't aware of how many harsh chemicals we are exposed to on a daily basis in our home-cleaning products. **One of the steps in leading a healthy life is to decrease or eliminate our exposure to all unnecessary chemicals**, which are toxic to both us and our environment. The first step can be in the kitchen with dish soaps. Today there are many alternatives. There are many environmentally friendly, hypoallergenic, dye- and perfume-free products available in health food stores and even some supermarkets. Words to look for: biodegradable, hypoallergenic, unscented, eco-friendly, non-chlorine bleaches, no animal testing (look for the bunny symbol).

Very Important: Please don't feel intimidated by anything that is written here. Take what feels right at first, and you'll see that as you walk the path, things that now seem totally unreasonable might feel comfortable later.

Remember: It is all about progress not perfe _____ (fill in the blank, refer to Step 3 "Staying In The Positive Zone", the quote list, on page 42.)

Step
4

What do you remember from this chapter? From everything mentioned, choose one baby step that you will incorporate into your life. Once you feel comfortable with that step, then choose another.

What will it be? When will you do it?

Getting Acquainted With Your Kitchenware

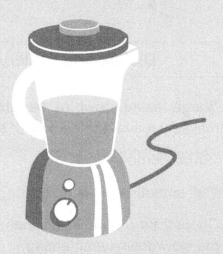

*With the right tools,
you're halfway there...*

Anonymous

Okay. Having covered some basic background, it's now time to check that you have the right basic kitchen equipment (your healthy "*tools*"). This will shorten your time in the kitchen and make cooking much healthier and easier. Most things can be bought in a household appliance store. Important "tools" are marked with an asterisk(*). As we go through the program you will understand their importance.

Dishes and Cutlery

☐ *Large salad bowl (a beautiful one that makes you want to eat lots of salad)

☐ *Small porridge bowl

☐ *Tall smoothie glass and a long spoon

☐ Chopsticks (I love using them – they help me slow down when eating)

Cooking Pots and Utensils

☐ *Pressure cooker (great for shortening kitchen time)

☐ Pots – in various sizes (note that Teflon non-stick pans and pots are very unhealthy, releasing different chemicals into the food, especially when they scratch so easily. Use stainless steel, cast iron, glass or ceramic.)

☐ Large pot (I place it in the sink, fill it with water and throw all the veggies in. It's a great way to wash them easily.)

☐ Pyrex oven baking dishes – in various sizes

☐ *3 good knives – large chopping, medium slicing, small paring

☐ Long cooking spoon

☐ Spatula (a very important tool when you are making a smoothie)

☐ Metal steamer basket (it's great to simply steam vegetables, like sweet potatoes, broccoli, cauliflower, or carrots, and eat them with olive oil and soy sauce.)

☐ Strainer (can be used for sprouting)

☐ Small sieve (I use it for rinsing dried fruit, cacao nibs, lentils.)

☐ Peeler (though I eat vegetables with the peel on, I love peeling strips of carrots and cucumbers straight into a salad.)

☐ Grater (it is good to grate carrots and beets into a salad; also for grating ginger.)

☐ Hand juicer (mostly for fresh lemon juice)

Appliances

☐ *Blender (preferably a very strong professional one, but a home type will work, too)

☐ Coffee grinder (to grind cacao nibs, chia seeds, flax seeds and spices)

☐ Juicer (for those who like juicing)

☐ Hand blender (great for creaming soups)

Other Items

- [ ] *Plastic or stainless steel box or flask (to take food to work or on the go)

- [ ] *Ice cube trays

- [ ] Large Ziploc bag (for storing nori packages in the freezer)

- [ ] Glass jars (for storing refrigerated nuts, legumes, seeds and whole grains, spices, other foodstuffs and leftovers – keeps them fresher)

- [ ] Lettuce dryer (water on lettuce and other greens makes the salad "tired," so I always dry lettuce and other greens. I often wash a variety of greens and store them refrigerated in the lettuce dryer, so when I want to make a salad everything is washed and ready to go.)

- [ ] Timer (so you don't have to stand near the food when it is cooking)

- [ ] Lazy Susan base (Place on your dinner table with different sauces and condiments so everyone can easily reach to flavor their own dish.)

Step
5

You don't have to get everything all at once. Check the list for what you already have and see if you can buy or even borrow the things you don't. As we continue the program and at your leisure, slowly get what you need.

Remember: The most important "vitamin" is to have fun while getting healthier.

Introductory Meeting With New Ingredients and a Health Food Store Tour

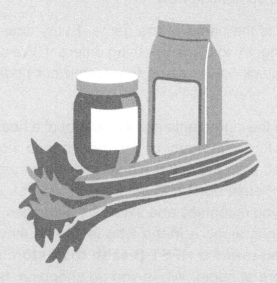

*Eat healthy food, have a healthy body.
This is the law of nature.*

S.N. Goenka

Once you have stocked up on some of the healthy ingredients, you very soon will become accustomed to reaching for them instead of using those that are unhealthy. It is important to have healthy alternatives at home so you have convenient and available options. That is the secret! Otherwise you automatically go to the unhealthy foods you are used to. You don't have to buy all of these at once, but every shopping trip you can add something new.

Variety is the name of the game. Every time you go shopping, try to buy something different. We all seem to get stuck on the same foods, and our bodies love variety.

Most of the ingredients can be bought at a health food store. I know for many of you, health food stores are like a strange unknown planet with weird unfamiliar foods. Please don't feel intimidated. At first, buy the things you recognize and slowly try new ones. Ask for help, bring along a friend who is into healthy eating and read over the **HFST (health food store tips)** to feel more at home. When you go shopping, take this helpful list with you.

Greens

☐ lettuce varieties	☐ kale
☐ parsley	☐ beet greens
☐ coriander	☐ dill
☐ celery	☐ mint
☐ spinach	☐ arugula
☐ basil	☐ broccoli
☐ mangold	☐ cabbage
(swiss chard)	☐ green onion

☀ HFST:

Greens are the most important food missing in people's diet nowadays. Make sure the greens are fresh, that the green color is bright and not turning yellow. Smell them – close your eyes and take a deep breath; feel nature flowing through your veins.

Sprouts

☐ alfalfa	☐ mung bean
☐ bean varieties	☐ radish
☐ chickpea	☐ broccoli
☐ lentil	

💡 HFST:

Sprouts are a little bundle of life force. When a grain or seed sprouts, the percentages of vitamins, enzymes, antioxidants, proteins and available sugars grow dramatically; sprouts are great to add to different dishes.

Vegetables	
☐ tomato	☐ red cabbage
☐ cucumber	☐ zucchini
☐ red pepper	☐ squash

💡 HFST:

Buy different colors of veggies; think of painting a rainbow with your food. Each color has different nutrients and health properties; the dark red and purple ones are full of anti-oxidants; the whites are like nature's pharmacy (onion, garlic), the orange are loaded with beta carotene. Think bright colors.

Sweet/ root vegetables	
☐ sweet potato	☐ carrot
☐ onion	☐ pumpkin
☐ celery root	

HFST:

These are great for balancing sugar cravings, very grounding. (See Step 18 "A Few More Tips For A Powerful Life", Grounding, on page 248.)

Whole grains

- [ ] quinoa (red, black, or white – the white is actually a bit refined, but still great)
- [ ] millet
- [ ] whole grain rice (long grain, short grain, red)
- [ ] black rice
- [ ] wheat berries
- [ ] rolled oats (big and flat, not the quick instant kind)
- [ ] buckwheat (actually a seed but we eat it as a grain)

HFST:

Pick one and try it. For a breakfast food, rolled oats are a great choice; for lunch or dinner, try quinoa – it takes only 20 minutes to cook.

Fruits

- ☐ apple
- ☐ banana
- ☐ melon
- ☐ papaya
- ☐ watermelon
- ☐ orange
- ☐ mandarin

- ☐ pomelo
- ☐ grapefruit
- ☐ pear
- ☐ mango
- ☐ berries
- ☐ grapes

 HFST:

Fruits are a great sweet treat and are delicious in smoothies.

Dried fruits

- ☐ figs
- ☐ dates

- ☐ raisins
- ☐ prunes

 HFST:

Dried fruits are another great sweet treat. You can eat them with nuts, or they are great in porridge. Eat in moderation since they do have a high sugar content.

Nuts

- ☐ brazil (high in selenium – has a strong anti-cancer effect)
- ☐ walnut (high in Omega 3, great for the brain – and they actually look like the brain)
- ☐ cashew (high in protein)
- ☐ almond (high in protein and calcium)
- ☐ pecan (high in iron)
- ☐ hazel
- ☐ macadamia

💡 **HFST:**

Nuts are a great source of proteins and healthy oils; each nut has different health properties. They are good to add to porridge or salads, or eat with fresh or dried fruit.

Legumes

- ☐ mung beans
- ☐ lentils (orange, yellow, green)
- ☐ adzuki
- ☐ chickpea
- ☐ lima

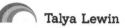

 HFST:

Legumes are a great vegetarian protein source, wonderful in soups, stews and salads. (I will teach you how to cook them for easy digestion – See Step 16 "Legumes & Sprouting" on page 213.)

Spices	
☐ cumin	☐ cayenne
☐ cinnamon	☐ Himalayan salt
☐ turmeric	☐ pepper

 HFST:

Buy organic spices if possible; these are great for adding flavor to salads, soups, stews and other dishes. Use in combinations, instead of using ready-mixed seasonings that are usually full of taste enhancers, MSG, salt and sugar.

Seeds	
☐ flax	☐ sunflower
☐ pumpkin	

HFST:

Seeds are great to add to salads, sandwiches and many other dishes.

Flavorings

☐ non-GMO soy sauce
☐ ginger root
☐ garlic
☐ juice and zest of lemon and citrus

☐ apple cider vinegar
☐ balsamic vinegar

Oils

☐ olive
☐ coconut

☐ sesame
☐ hemp

 HFST:

Buy organic, extra-virgin, first cold-pressed oils, in a dark glass bottle or metal can.

Seaweeds

☐ arame   ☐ wakame
☐ dulse   ☐ hijiki
☐ nori   ☐ kombu (kelp)

🔆 HFST:

These are usually found in the Asian section; each package has instructions on how to use them. They are great for adding flavor and minerals to salads, soups, stews and other dishes, help to balance salt cravings and are great for the hair and skin. (Caution: If you have a hyperthyroid condition it is better not to eat seaweed.)

Others

☐ tahini and other nut   ☐ olives
  pastes (besides   ☐ dark chocolate
  peanut butter)   (at least 70
☐ sardines in olive oil   percent cacao)

HFST:

Dark chocolate is a great healthy snack that crowds out the unhealthy snacks. Look for organic, with no soy, milk, white sugar or preservatives.

Superfoods

- ☐ goji berries
- ☐ mulberries
- ☐ cacao beans and nibs
- ☐ maca powder
- ☐ bee pollen
- ☐ hulled hemp seeds and hemp powder

- ☐ spirulina
- ☐ chia seeds
- ☐ kelp powder
- ☐ chlorela
- ☐ barley grass
- ☐ wheatgrass
- ☐ carob powder

See Step 7 "Upgrade Yourself With Superfoods" on page 87.

Sweeteners

- [ ] real raw honey (unheated and unpasteurized)
- [ ] maple syrup grade B
- [ ] Xylitol
- [ ] silan
- [ ] date sugar
- [ ] organic cane sugar
- [ ] molasses

HFST:

Use these healthier options to crowd out unhealthy sweeteners like white sugar and artificial sweeteners. They are usually located together.

Other Important Tips for Shopping

- **Not everything** that is in a health food store **is healthy**.

- **Be a food detective**. Question what is inside the package; don't just believe the slogans like *natural, healthy, pure, whole grains, organic, free-range.*

- **Read food labels**. Buy products with ingredients you can pronounce and identify; it is also better to buy foods that don't have more than five or six ingredients listed. Ingredients are listed in descending order of amounts, so the first few ingredients at the top of the list are found in the largest amounts in that food. If sugar, vegetable oil (which is usually margarine), white flour and salt are listed at the beginning, those are the main ingredients in what you are eating. I try to stay away from foods that have sugar and vegetable oil in the ingredient list. Once you start reading you will notice that salt and sugar are in all processed packaged foods. (Sugar has many different names: table sugar, sucrose, powdered sugar, brown sugar, lactose, dextrose, glucose, HFCS, high fructose corn syrup, corn syrup, sorbitol.)

• **Stay away from anything that says diet, low-fat or low-calorie.** These foods are loaded with artificial sweeteners, other chemicals, salt and all kinds of stuff you don't want to be eating. They also make you eat more than you would have had you been eating the real thing. They make you gain weight. Our bodies have been designed to eat food, not things that look like food but aren't really.

When I studied health counseling in New York City, one of our teachers, Marion Nestle, explained why we should stay away from the middle aisles of typical supermarkets. She explained that most supermarkets are designed pretty much the same. Fruits and vegetables at the entrance – to make us feel like this is a healthy place, a market. At the back you have the dairy products; since many people come just to get a carton of milk or some cheese, they will have to go through the whole supermarket to get it, and the more you see the more you buy. On the sides are the fish and meat counters. And in the middle are rows and rows of processed unhealthy foods. When you enter an aisle, there is no way out. You have to go to the end, and you will probably pick up a few items along the way. So try to stay out of the middle aisles.

Step
6

Tick off what you already have from the list, and after reading the next chapter or next few chapters, if you feel ready to cook something (which is of course simple, delicious and healthy), decide on a few ingredients to buy.

Check if there is a health food store in your area.

Remember: Smile. Breathe. Be stress-free. Be calm. Be happy. Be cool.

Everything is happening exactly as it should.

You are so cool. You are so cool.
You are so cool.

"True Romance," Tarantino

Upgrade Yourself With Superfoods

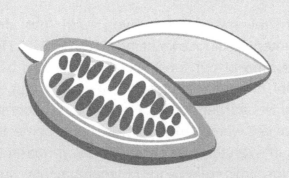

*Let food be thy medicine
and medicine be thy food.*

Hippocrates

When I was a kid growing up, we listened to LP records. In the early '80s my family moved for two years to Zaire (now the Democratic Republic of the Congo) in Africa. My parents bought an enormous radio, and we were able to listen to the news from Israel. For my 15th birthday, I was given a large radio-tape recorder. Later I got a small Walkman, and a few years after that I upgraded to a Discman. Now, we all have tiny little iPods, iPhones, iPads … none of us is using the same computer we started with.

Don't get me wrong. Even with our improved equipment, I still love listening to the old LPs. However, in the area of our food, instead of it also becoming smaller but better and better, it seems that the very opposite has happened. Foods have become much bigger yet worse and worse. Foods come in super sizes in everything, but with far fewer nutrients, fiber, vitamins, minerals and phytochemicals, and with many more toxic substances: saturated oils, refined sugar and salt, artificial chemicals, lab-created vitamins, heavy metals, pesticides and herbicides.

In the USA today, two-thirds of the population are obese or on their way there, one out of three young people are overweight and kids have adult-onset diabetes. There is an epidemic of global obesity; more and more people have cancer, heart problems, depression, diabetes. The U.S. politician Mike Huckabee said, "We are digging our graves with our knife and fork."

How Do You Upgrade Your Food?

Eating healthily doesn't mean that you stop enjoying food. On the contrary! You choose a healthier, upgraded version of what you love. Doesn't it seem reasonable that if we put natural, organic, healthy foods into our body, it will have an effect on our moods, energy, thoughts, happiness, health, awareness and overall quality of life?

 Secret Tips:

Place your **focus on what is healthy and what you can choose** – not on what you are "missing out on."

Most people don't know this: **the higher the quality – the lower the quantity**. The higher the quality of the food you eat, the lower the quantity you need. And it works in the opposite direction, too: the lower the quality of the food you eat, the more you will eat. When eating high-quality food, naturally and easily, you also lose weight. People try to lose weight by eating diet/low-calorie foods that only make them eat more.

Eat the real thing and forget about the calories:

- Eat healthy oils (olive and coconut oils, nuts, seeds, avocados, whole coconut) instead of oil-free.

- Eat avocado (even though it is said to be fattening) and forget about low-calorie cheese.

- Eat a handful of nuts and dried fruit instead of a low-calorie snack bar.

- Eat fruit instead of diet cookies.

- Eat good quality bread – instead of diet bread or rice crackers (those crackers never seem to fill me anyway).

> Stay away from anything that has diet, low-calorie or low-fat written on it. It isn't real food, is loaded with all kinds of artificial and unhealthy ingredients and it will make YOU low and fat.

Superfoods

One of the best and easiest ways to upgrade the quality of your food is to add superfoods (superfuels) to your diet. You don't have to change anything; all you have to do is add them to what already is.

I have been eating healthily for years and, on and off, a vegetarian diet. A few years back, while I was eating a healthy vegan, fruit, vegetable, nuts and seeds, grain diet, I realized I wasn't doing that well: I was losing hair, my nails were breaking, I was craving sweets (even though I ate healthy sweets, I was eating too many apples, dates and organic dark chocolate), and my brain wasn't functioning in the way I knew it should. And then, while studying nutrition at IIN, David Wolfe the raw food superfood "guru" gave us a rock and roll, life-transforming lecture. I learned about superfoods. I was very inspired and right away started adding them to my diet.

Well – there really is no other way to say it: It was **life-transforming**. Since adding superfoods to my diet, I have never felt better. I have never felt happier. I have tons of energy and focus, my digestion is like a Swiss clock, my hair is thick, my nails are strong, my brain is doing the job and I have no more cravings for sweets. I still eat healthy sweets, but in a balanced way and in smaller amounts.

THE POWER OF ADDING

Overcome Sugar Cravings and Other Issues with Superfoods

One of my clients in his late 30s came to me with digestive problems, gas, bloating, constipation, horrible sweet cravings (he ate about three chocolate bars a day), frequent sickness and low energy. He didn't want to stop having coffee, pizza, pasta and sweets. So all we did was add superfoods to his diet. He incorporated a superfood smoothie once a day and added lots of superfoods to his porridge that he was already eating. Six months have gone by. He feels really healthy. His digestive problems are gone. After two weeks of drinking the smoothie, he said he had no desire to eat any more chocolate. He still has one coffee a day and every now and then a pizza. But all in all, thanks to superfoods, he has upgraded his life naturally and easily.

What Are Superfoods?

These are real foods. They are not supplements; they are not created in a lab by scientists; they are highly concentrated in nutrients and have been consumed by native peoples in various parts of the world for thousands of years. Adding them to your daily diet can be transforming. Have one superfood smoothie a day, and you may get more nutrients than the average person gets in one week. Add them to your porridge, and feel the difference in your energy level, health, focus, mood, digestion and more!

Don't take my word for it. It isn't about believing what I say! **It is about you trying it out for yourself** – and seeing what it does for **YOU**. Try it for a month. Once you feel the difference, you won't dream of going back to that slow old computer.

Superfoods have unusual, exotic names and new flavors, but when you and your body get used to them, it will seem like you have been eating them forever.

Start by incorporating some that are accessible and then slowly add in a few more at a time. Eat them raw (uncooked), so they keep all their amazing nutrients.

What do you do with them? You'll just have to continue to the next chapter. But first, here is a list of a few superfoods that I use on a daily basis; I recommend starting off with these.

Bee Pollen

Flowers produce this powder and honeybees collect it. It is a rich source of high-quality protein, contains all essential amino acids, is great for the brain and is loaded with minerals, vitamins and enzymes. Try to purchase bee products from smaller, local hives, since it is very important that the bees are treated with respect and in a humane way and not as they are in the large commercial industrial hives.

If you are allergic to bees, make sure you aren't allergic to pollen, too. It is available in small granules and has a sweet and unique flavor.

 Tip:

I buy raw bee pollen. It is found in the freezer section and should also be transported to the store under refrigeration; at home, keep in the freezer.

How to use: 1-2 teaspoons in a smoothie, on porridge, organic goat yogurt, granola, on a salad or eat just as it is.

Cacao Beans/ Nibs/ Powder

Great for chocoholics, this is the bean/ seed of the cacao fruit. Real chocolate is made from cacao beans.

Cacao is the best source of magnesium (the most deficient mineral in people's diets) and contains many other minerals like iron, calcium, zinc and chromium (stabilizes blood sugar levels). Raw cacao, which hasn't been heated over 48 degrees Celsius, has high levels of antioxidants (much more than red wine and green tea). Cacao balances brain chemistry, is great for the heart and brain, is a natural laxative (due to the high magnesium levels) and is a hormone balancer.

Overall, cacao beans give us amazing energy and make us feel happy (by raising our serotonin levels) and relaxed. To taste the full flavor, first put a raw cacao bean (or nibs) in a teaspoon with a bit of honey, maple syrup or any other natural sweetener and eat it like that – it tastes like dark bitter chocolate. Now take another bean, put it in your mouth, suck on it and chew it very slowly, letting all the flavors explode. It is a little bitter, but that is what real cacao tastes like.

 Tip:

Cacao is available in beans, nibs or powder. I prefer the nibs or beans. I would like to emphasize that cacao, though one of my favorites, isn't beneficial for everyone. It is best eaten in moderation. Carry some cacao beans or nibs with you. If you need an energy boost, instead of going for a sugar rush or coffee, try some cacao with goji berries, mulberries or dried fruit.

How to use: 1-2 teaspoons in a smoothie, on porridge, organic goat yogurt or granola, on a salad or with a little honey, maple syrup or a date, or just eat it by itself.

Chia Seeds

These are extremely high in Omega-3 fatty acids (600 percent more than salmon) and loaded with antioxidants, vitamins, minerals and fiber. They are high in calcium (higher calcium content than milk) and protein. They are great for lubricating the system and preventing constipation. They are also great little energy boosters; they used to be called "the running food," since runners of the Inca people would eat a handful and run for the whole day on the energy they gave.

Tip:

Available in whole or ground seeds.

How to use: Throw some into your water bottle and just sip them all day long. Put 1-2 teaspoons in a smoothie, on porridge, organic goat yogurt, or a salad.

You can make raw dehydrated crackers from them. Their unique biological properties aren't ruined by heat; therefore chia can be used in baking, too. It is best to pre-soak – they will expand tremendously, about 10 times.

Goji Berries

These are called Red Diamonds in the Far East – the Goji power!!! It is a berry that originally grew in the Himalayas and has been the No. 1 food/ herb in Chinese Medicine for over 6,000 years. Goji berries are a great source of vegetarian protein, with eighteen amino acids, more than 20 different minerals, vitamins (including vitamin C), beta carotene and antioxidants. They stimulate the body to produce the growth hormone (HGH), so they are also "anti-aging." You can start off by tossing some onto your salad or by eating them as a snack with some nuts.

 Tip:

Available in whole berries or powder – I prefer the whole berry.

How to use: put 1 tablespoon in a smoothie, add to porridge, organic goat yogurt, granola, desserts and salads, or eat with a few nuts or cacao nibs for a healthy snack.

Hemp Seeds/ Powder/ Oil

This is one of my favorite superfoods! No worries, the products from this variety will not mess with your psyche.

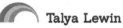
Hemp food products (hulled hemp seeds, hemp protein powder, hemp milk) are made from the cannabis sativa plant, which has many amazing nutritious qualities. The hemp plant that is smoked and has high amounts of THC (tetrahydrocannabinol – the psychoactive drug) comes from a different variety.

Hemp is one of nature's most perfect plants. It can grow almost anywhere, without the use of pesticides or fertilizers, and is therefore healthy for the environment. The hemp seed is extremely high in protein (about 33 percent), contains all eight essential amino acids and more Edestin (a bioactive protein that is very easy to digest) than any other plant. It is also high in chlorophyll, essential fatty acids, magnesium, iron and zinc. It is the king of all superfoods.

> *If people let government decide what foods they eat and what medicines they take, their bodies will soon be in as sorry a state as are the souls of those who live under tyranny.*
>
> Thomas Jefferson

Tip:

Hemp is available in seeds, powder, milk or oil. The seeds and powder are great for those who want to build muscle. Just have some hemp after your workout and ditch those toxic protein powders full of soy, whey, sugar and taste enhancers.

How to use: The powder can be mixed into smoothies, juice or just water. Use the hulled seeds in smoothies, porridge, organic goat yogurt, granola, desserts or salads. The oil is great in smoothies and salads, but don't heat it and keep it refrigerated.

Maca Powder

I love it! Read about it and try it and you will love it, too. Maca is a Peruvian root vegetable from the radish family. It has been used since the time of the Incas as both a food and a medicine. It is great for balancing the thyroid, balancing hormones, boosting fertility and treating menstrual disorders, menopause symptoms. It is known to increase memory and focus, to promote emotional well-being and to work as an anti-depressant. It also is a great energy booster and an aphrodisiac!

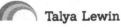

 Tip:

Available in powder. If you eat it daily, it is recommended to go off it every month for one week. A little break makes the body "miss" it and may enhance its effectiveness.

How to use: 1 teaspoon in a smoothie, porridge or organic goat yogurt, or mix in water.

Seaweed

I love seaweed. I use several kinds on a daily base: I put the powdered ones (spirulina, chlorella, kelp) in my smoothies and others (dulse, wakame, hijiki, arame, kombo, nori) in salads and warm dishes. And I use the nori for making rolls.

Seaweeds are one of the most nutritionally dense foods. They are loaded with minerals: calcium, iron, iodine, potassium. They can have between 10-20 more minerals than earth vegetables have, especially since today the land is very depleted. They have high amounts of vitamins (some even have vitamin B12, so they are great for vegetarians), protein and more. They can also:

- Boost your metabolism

- Supply high qantities of iodine, an essential mineral

for healthy thyroid function

- Help stabilize hormones

- Aid in lowering cholesterol

- Strengthen the hair, skin and nails

Note: If you suffer from hyperthyroidism, you shouldn't include seaweeds in your diet. Here's more on specific seaweeds.

Spirulina

A tiny single-celled blue-green algae, spirulina is a seaweed and one of the most nutrient-dense foods available. It is a concentrated, easily digestible source of complete protein (at least 65 percent is protein), so for example one teaspoon of spirulina has the same amount of protein as 36 grams of beef. It is great for blood purification, has anti-inflammatory and joint strengthening properties and is high in antioxidants. It is a great energy booster.

 Tip:

Available in powder or dried leaves.

How to use: Start off with 1/4 teaspoon and gradually increase to 1-2 teaspoons a day, depending on your taste and digestion. Add to smoothies, soups, salads or energy bars.

Kelp (kombo)

This algae (seaweed) contains high levels of iodine and is great for thyroid function. It is very potent, so 1/4 teaspoon a day is likely to be enough for most people. Put a 10-centimeter piece in stews and soups (don't worry, it won't interfere with the flavor).

 Tip:

Available in powder or whole seaweed leaves.

Chlorella

This algae is great for purifying the blood from toxins and heavy metals and for lowering cholesterol. A flat teaspoon a day should be enough for most people.

 Tip:

Available in powder and tablets (make sure the tablets don't have any binding agents).

Hijiki/ Wakame/ Arame

Soak in cold water for about 20-30 minutes, squeeze

out the water and mix in salads and other dishes. Use the water on your plants or give to your pet (it is high in minerals).

Nori

Cut into salads or use for making sushi. In the upcoming chapter *My Basic Summer Meal*, I will teach you exactly what I do with it!

Step
7

We have just covered a lot of information.

Remember: Health is a journey – not a destination.

Break the journey down into small baby steps.

There are many more superfoods, but I don't want you to become overwhelmed. I suggest starting off with a couple and seeing how you react. Once you start feeling comfortable, you can investigate and add more.

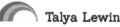

Choose one or two superfoods to start with.

Which will they be?

When will you buy them?

You can find most of the superfoods in health food stores or you may place an order over the web. There are many good companies on the market.

For further information on this subject, I also recommend looking into David Wolfe's work, one of the leading world authorities on raw food and super-foods. His books include *Naked Chocolate, Super-foods: The Food and Medicine of the Future and The Sunfood Diet Success System*.

Please continue to the next chapter for some simple ideas on how to incorporate superfoods into your diet.

The So Very Important Breakfast

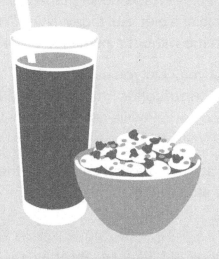

*This is your life,
not a dress rehearsal.*

Jim Donovan

When I was in high school in the late 1980s, it was all about counting calories. I don't know how I did it, but for breakfast I would have a little rice cracker with two tablespoons of cottage cheese, a few slices of tomato and a splash of olive oil. At school I would drink Diet Coke and have one large green apple. That was it until I got home around two or three and had a low-calorie lunch. Shocking for me now, don't you think?! God only knows how I managed to think at all with that kind of a diet. But today, NO WAY JOSÉ! You won't catch me without a nutritious breakfast.

What about you? Do you eat breakfast? What do you have? Is it a cup of coffee in the car on the way to work? Some boxed cereal while reading the newspaper?

Many people skip breakfast, because they are too busy, they are trying to cut calories or they had a late dinner and are still digesting it.

> **I would like to emphasize this**: For most people, breakfast is the most important meal of the day.

The word "breakfast" actually refers to breaking the fast of the night. It is like regulating the thermostat of our body, and the way we start our day influences our whole day. Compare starting the day with a cup of coffee and a cookie on the go, or taking 20 minutes in the morning to sit calmly and have something nutritious to eat. I hear you saying, "I don't have time." Well, I will not accept that. Make time!

> You owe it to yourself. It is your born right. Don't let anything come between you and your breakfast!

The minute you turn it into a habit, you won't understand how you lived without it. We are creatures of habit – we can get used to anything. And as far as the calories go, research shows that people who eat breakfast consume overall fewer calories in a day than people who skip it and get to lunch starving. Anyway, it is much healthier to have most of your food during the first half of the day (breakfast and lunch) and less for dinner.

We are all different. Some do well with a light breakfast (like fruit), while others need something heavier, but no matter what you do, don't have a cup of coffee on an empty stomach. If you need coffee, have it after a meal as a digestive aid. Beginning your day with coffee is like going to the bank every day and taking out $5 when you are already in the red.

This is how I start the day:

- First thing in the morning, after cleaning my tongue and brushing my teeth (check the tongue scraper in Step 18 "A Few More Tips For A Powerful Life" on page 252), I have a large glass of lukewarm water with (or without) some freshly squeezed lemon juice from half a lemon. I sometimes eat an orange or pomela with it, too.

- I take my dog for a ten-minute walk.

- I have a shower, do a few stretches.

- I eat my breakfast.

As I said earlier, make time. The breakfast options presented here are really easy and shouldn't take very long to prepare, especially the smoothie, which is the easiest thing – everyone has time for a smoothie. If you aren't hungry for breakfast, check if that is your nature. Or are you eating your dinner too late the night before?

Here are some easy *Breaking the Fast* options:

My Favorite Green Super(Food) Smoothie

This is my recommended healthiest spring/ summer breakfast. Everyone has time to make this smoothie. All you need is a blender, some fruit, green leaves and superfoods. You don't need to have all the ingredients on the list, just start with whatever you can find. A smoothie is so easy to make. You can feed the whole family in 10 minutes. It is not only delicious, but it gives you loads of energy and nutrition. Even if you think you need to chew to feel satisfied, give it a try and make it thick. "Eat" it with a long spoon from a tall glass, and see how you get "addicted" to it. It becomes the best part of the day. When you go to sleep you will wish it was already morning.

I actually don't measure anything but just throw different ingredients into the blender and add a bit of this and that until it tastes yummy. So the amounts are just approximations. Play around with it until you find your recipe. Even if the first one isn't delicious, don't give up. Eventually you will master the art of making your perfect Super Smoothie.

Smoothie

Ingredients - for 1 smoothie:

- Superfoods (goji, chia, cacao, hemp, spirulina, bee pollen)

- Fruit (1 very ripe banana + ¾ cup other fruit)

- Leafy greens (swiss chard, mint, kale, spinach) – I use the whole leaf (stems, too)

- Coconut oil (1 tablespoon cold-pressed)

- Ice (if you live in a cold climate or in wintertime, you can skip the ice)

- Water (I don't put too much, ½ - ¾ cup, since I like a thicker consistency)

Directions:

If your blender is a really strong, professional one, you can blend everything at once. Put the ingredients straight into the blender, and you barely have to cut anything. I recommend adding the ice cubes at the end, after everything is blended, and then blend a bit more, otherwise the coconut oil will harden.

»

If your blender is of normal household strength, it is better to put ingredients in gradually. You might want to soak the gojis together with the chia in some water in a separate bowl for a few minutes before blending them, and take the stems off the green leaves.

Here is how I make my smoothie:

- Soak 1 teaspoon chia seeds straight in the blender

- In a tall smoothie glass, melt the coconut oil with a little boiling water

- Add to the blender: 1 very ripe banana (the riper, the sweeter) and 3/4 cup of either melon, grapes, mango, papaya, pineapple, berries or any other fruit (or a combination of two)

- Add some leafy greens: mint (3-6 stems), 1-2 swiss chard or 1 kale leaf or a bunch of spinach. At the beginning go easy on the greens; as you get used to them and to their flavor, you can use more.

- Teaspoons: 1-2 raw cacao nibs, ½-1 carob powder, 1 spirulina*, 1 maca**.

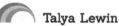

- 1 tablespoon bee pollen, goji berries, hulled hemp seeds (or hemp powder)

- Add a little more water if needed and blend, increasing the speed gradually

- Pour in the melted coconut while the blender is still running and blend till very smooth

- Add a few ice cubes (you don't want to make it too cold – in winter I skip the ice but in warm weather you may add more ice as it is nice to drink chilled)

- Pour into a tall glass and eat/ drink slowly using a long spoon.

- Chew it, mix it with your saliva and have a Super New Day!

- Use the spatula from the food equipment list to scrape out the remaining smoothie in the blender. It is actually the best part!

---

* Start off with 1/4 teaspoon and every few days gradually increase the amount. It takes a while to get used to the taste and allow your body to create the enzymes to digest it.

** Maca is a Peruvian root vegetable from the radish family that increases resistance to stress and balances endocrine hormones and the immune system (actually helps the body adapt to the stress of modern life – an adaptogen).

Remember: Don't believe me, but try it yourself and observe what happens in your body, energy level and mind, in just one week. You have to experience it and find out the truth, whether or not it works for you.

Let me show you how quick it is – it takes less time than boiling water in the kettle.

Smoothie – Superlife's Healthy Habit Program

Tips:

- Soak the chia seeds in water before putting them in the smoothie.

- Rinse the goji berries and cacao nibs in a small sieve.

- Add more water if you prefer a more liquid consistency.

- Add more ice cubes if you prefer it colder.

- Start off with fewer greens and add more when you get used to the flavor. It is recommended to rotate your greens, trying out different ones.

- If needed you can sweeten with honey, maple syrup or 1-2 dates (but if the fruit is very ripe, you won't have to).

- Switch around and add other superfoods: refer to Step 7 "Upgrade Yourself With Superfoods" on page 87 for ideas (adding a vanilla bean or powder is very delicious).

- Make sure your smoothie has more than just fruit. You need some oil (like coconut oil, hemp oil, avocado or nuts – cashews make the smoothie very smooth) or some high-protein superfoods (like bee pollen, hemp, spirulina, maca) to slow down the absorption of the sugar and keep you satisfied for several hours.

How to Clean the Blender in 15 Seconds?

People always tell me that cleaning the blender takes up most of the time. It is actually so easy. Fill ¾ full with warm water, a bit of soap and turn on high for 15 seconds. Magic – it's done!

My Delicious Comforting Super(Food) Porridge

This is my recommended healthiest winter-time breakfast. Eat this instead of eating boxed cereals devoid of any live energy, that can sit for months if not years on the supermarket shelf without anything happening to them. Even though they may say whole grain, natural, vitamins and minerals added (which actually are synthetic, unhealthy and petroleum-based), switch-up to this delicious porridge dish. It is really easy! And great for cold winter days.

> **Remember**: You want to eat food that has live energy in it and not foods that are man-laboratory-made, pumped with all kinds of synthetic vitamins and preservatives.

Porridge

Ingredients – for 1 serving:

- 1/2 cup of whole oats (minimally processed with only the outer hull removed, larger, not the pre-cooked, instant, quick, small size kind)

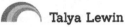
- Coconut oil, raisins, cinnamon, nuts, tahini, fruit

- Superfoods: hulled hempseeds, cacao nibs, goji, chia, mulberries, bee pollen

Directions:

1. The night before, soak 1/2 cup of oats in a pot filled with water to cover. This neutralizes the phytic acid in the grains, which prohibits absorption of minerals in the body.

2. In the morning cook soaked oats on a low flame for about 7-10 minutes in the soaking water (no need to change the water) until the consistency is the way you like it. I make my porridge in water; I don't use milk. Stir from time to time – add more water if needed. I add quite a lot of water as I like it liquidy, since it thickens as it cools when all the other goodies are added.

3. To save on time, while the porridge is cooking, soak (in a bit of hot or cold water) 1-2 teaspoons of chia, some raisins, a teaspoon of cacao nibs, goji berries, other superfoods.

»

4. Put some porridge in the bowl, add cinnamon (balances sugar levels) and mix well (if you are making the exact amount you will eat, you can mix it all in the pot).

5. Put some coconut oil on top (in the winter the oil is hard and will melt), slice a banana, sprinkle some walnuts (great source of Omega 3 fatty acids) and a bit of tahini. You can also sweeten with silan, honey or maple syrup.

I like to eat it with a long spoon, enjoying each mouthful.

Let me show you how quick it is.

Porridge Breakfast – Superlife's Healthy Habit Program

 Tips:

• You can rinse the goji berries, cacao nibs and raisins in a small sieve.

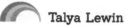

- Use other superfoods, fruits, dried fruits and nuts.

- You can add superfoods as long as you don't cook them (you may cook the chia, as its unique biological properties are not diminished by heat).

- If you've made extra, cool the rest and keep in the fridge for eating in the next few days.

- Every day you can warm just enough for each meal (in a small pot with a little water).

A Salty Mediterranean Porridge Option

Ingredients – for 1 serving:

- Cooked porridge

- Vegetables (I like tomatoes and cucumbers)

- Leafy greens (I like parsley or coriander)

- Black olives

- Cumin powder

- Olive oil

>>

Directions:

1. Put warm or cool porridge in a bowl, add some cut greens and mix together.

2. On top, slice a cucumber, tomato, some more cut greens, and add a few olives.

3. Sprinkle with cumin and pour olive oil generously on top.

4. Eat with a long spoon, enjoying each bite.

Buckwheat Breakfast

This is another great breakfast. Buckwheat is very high in protein, gluten-free and mild in taste. Use the green unroasted one.

Even if you think you don't like buckwheat – you have to try this recipe.

Ingredients – for 1 serving:

- 1/2 cup unroasted buckwheat (soak overnight)

- almond milk – so easy to make your own

>>

(see recipe on page 121)

- superfoods (cacao nibs, chia seeds, goji berries)
- cinnamon
- optional: nuts, raisins, healthy granola
- strawberries

Directions:

1. Soak buckwheat overnight.

2. Rinse and cook in twice the amount of water for 10-15 minutes, till soft but still crunchy.

3. Strain off excess water and place in bowl.

4. Add nuts, raisins, superfoods, cinnamon.

5. Add almond milk.

6. Slice strawberries on top.

Buckwheat Porridge – Superlife's Healthy Habit Program

Easy Almond Milk

1. Soak a handful of almonds overnight.

2. In the morning drain and blend the almonds with a half-cup of water.

3. Strain.

4. Voila – you have almond milk!!

Or you can just blend water with almond paste.

Almond Milk – Superlife's Healthy Habit Program

Other Breakfast Ideas

- Salty options: whole grain toast with either avocado, tahini, goat cheese or an organic egg. To each, add olive oil, olives, vegetables and leafy greens.

- Sweet options: whole grain toast with tahini and honey (other options: maple syrup or date silan), you can also add coconut oil and cacao nibs. When the toast is warm, spread coconut oil generously on top, spread tahini and honey and sprinkle with cacao nibs – it is more delicious than cake!

- Fruit, or fruit with some nuts and other superfoods.

- Juice: here are two different juice options; cucumber, celery, fennel, carrot and beets; or carrots, green apples, ginger, orange juice or pomegranate juice (or half and half). You can also add spirulina and chlorella.

 Tips:

- In order to feel satisfied longer, eat carbs (like porridge, bread, fruit, dried fruit) together with proteins (nuts, seeds, chia seeds, goji berries, other high protein superfoods, eggs) and healthy oils.

- Don't think calories – think about having a healthy breakfast.

- Try to rotate your breakfast ingredients. Once you get into having the super smoothie or the super porridge, chances are you won't want to go for anything else, but rotate the greens and the fruit.

- See how you feel with different breakfasts and find

out what works best for your body type.

- Try to eat less at night so you wake up hungry.

- Consider it as your birthright to begin the day calmly with a nutritious breakfast.

Your Personal Lab Test

In order to follow the effects of what you are doing and the changes you are experiencing, to get the "lab" results from your body, I recommend filling in the chart below for the first week or so. On the first day have your regular breakfast (or not at all if you aren't accustomed to having breakfast), but still fill in the chart. On the following days try different breakfasts or repeat the same one, writing down each time how you feel: energy level, mood, happiness, hunger, digestion; did you snack less?

Find out what works best for your specific, special one-of-a-kind "machine." See how you feel right after eating, then 30 minutes later, 1-2 hours later. Rate it from 1-5. You can also do this chart for other meals and snacks. Your body will tell you exactly what is good for you.

Date	Breakfast time and food	How I feel right after	How I feel 1-2 hours after	Am I hungry for lunch?	Food cravings I had today

Step
8

Start with breakfast. It is a great and simple step.

You might not have to change much at all, only add some superfoods to what you are already eating. Or if you aren't accustomed to having breakfast, start to eat one, without superfoods, trying one of the options in this step.

Try to eat a smaller dinner, or eat dinner earlier. Even if you are accustomed to eating late, try gradually to eat dinner 15 minutes earlier.

Note: You can decide to stay with this step for a while before moving on to other steps. I really recommend you try to have some kind of a breakfast, and check how superfoods work for you. But if you choose to skip eating breakfast after all, skip this step and move on to the next.

Remember: Step by step. Baby steps. Little tiny steps. Simple steps. Have fun. Love yourself. You are doing great!

My Basic Summer Lunch Meal
A Few Life Changing Tips

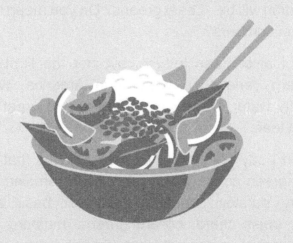

*Every blade of grass has its angel that bends
over it and whispers, "Grow, grow."*

The Talmud

I think this is one of the best discoveries ever! So buckle up and let's get started.

But before we begin, I have two questions for you:

1. What vegetables do you eat during the day?

2. Even more important, what leafy greens do you eat on a regular basis?

If you are like most people, the answer to the second question will be, "Leafy greens? Do you mean lettuce? And cucumbers?"

Yes, I also mean lettuce, but not the light-colored iceberg variety, so popular in America, which is mostly water. Cucumber is green and great but it's not a leaf...

When I say leafy greens I mean leaves that have a dark green color, full of chlorophyll: romaine lettuce, celery, parsley, coriander, mint, dill, basil, arugula, kale, swiss chard, collard greens, mustard greens, beet greens, green cabbage (though lighter in color), spinach, broccoli – there are so many. They are the most important food and most missed in our diets.

Supersize Your Salad

In the modern western world we have supersized the wrong foods.

Here comes your next step: From today on, I would like to suggest you **make your salad the main course at lunchtime** with lots of LEAFY GREENS (choose at least two besides lettuce) and everything else secondary.

> I want to emphasize that I am not suggesting to only eat a raw salad – certainly have other cooked foods with it – but make the salad big and give it the importance it deserves.

This works really well, especially for women. Some men do well with a big salad too, while others need to get used to it or prefer a smaller salad and some more substantial protein. Just make sure you have lots of fresh veggies and especially greens every day.

I love looking at people. I often watch what people order in restaurants. Though some people do eat a small salad with their meal, most don't have a salad at all or only have a few slices of tomato and a little iceberg lettuce. Try making the salad really big and significant. Now I'm not talking diet mentality here; it is not about counting calories or depriving yourself. I'm talking about adding living foods to your diet and making the salad the tastiest ever, the richest ever,

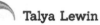
full of different colored vegetables, lots of greens, sprouts, seeds, seaweed, a delicious dressing (no diet dressings, no measuring oil with a teaspoon). Eventually you will get "addicted" to fresh vegetables and LEAFY GREENS, Nature's amazing gift to us. Then, add to it all the other foodstuffs, or rather place them all **on top** of the salad. The salad is the base.

Are You Asking, Why?

First, if you make a big, beautiful, colorful delicious salad and eat smaller portions of everything else, you will feel much better, lighter, more energetic and happier. I promise you! You won't have that post-meal feeling of heaviness you are often used to. And you might lose weight, too.

> **Food For Thought:** When you put gas in your car, does the car have to sleep and digest before it can go on?

Here are several more **reasons to consider**:

1. Greens Are a Superfood

What is the main food all big herbivore animals eat? What do giraffes, elephants, zebras, cows, rhinos, goats and chimpanzees eat? They all get their nutrients – minerals, vitamins, proteins – from lots of green leaves. Ever see a cow eat dairy for strong bones? Ever see a gorilla eat meat? But they do munch on leaves. That is because greens are loaded with all the good nutritional stuff. Of all foods, the LEAFY GREENS are nutritionally the most beneficial to our bodies! And we have 95 percent of the same genetic code as chimpanzees.

2. High in Protein

I hear you asking, "But what about proteins?" Well, one of the main sources of protein is LEAFY GREENS. Much more than other foods. Surprisingly, one of the foods many vegetarians miss out on is LEAFY GREENS.

3. Widest Health Benefits

LEAFY GREENS have great properties for preventing cancer, for supporting a healthy intestinal flora and purifying the blood, the liver and the kidneys. They are alkalizing, are full of antioxidants, aid in flexibility and much more.

4. High in Chlorophyll

Chlorophyll is the plant's "blood." It actually is sun energy that plants turn into something we can use. The structure of chlorophyll and hemoglobin are virtually the same, with only one difference: the main molecule of chlorophyll is magnesium, while the main molecule of our blood is iron. When we eat greens, the chlorophyll goes straight into our blood, purifying it.

5. Connect to Nature

Most of us are city people, breathing air very thin in oxygen. Take a look at a stalk of broccoli, a head of celery. Don't they look like little trees? Well, they are miniature trees. Put your nose in a fresh bunch of celery, parsley, basil ... close your eyes and take a deep breath – doesn't it feels like you are out in nature in a green field? City people especially need to eat greens, connect to nature, let oxygen flow in our veins.

6. Uplifting Energy

Even if we put aside all the health benefits of greens, let's look at their energy. Food isn't only calories, carbs, fats and proteins – food possesses energy. Each food has different energy. If you think about the nature of greens, they grow from the ground up to the sky: they have an uplifting energy. They grow up to the sun. Ever so many people today are heavy, down, low, depressed, popping anti-depressants. What about adding LEAFY GREENS to your diet and seeing how you feel? Try it and notice if energetically you feel a difference: lighter, happier, more creative.

Check out Victoria Boutenko's book, *Green for Life* for more information on Greens.

**Eat Your Greens – Superlife's
Healthy Habit Program**

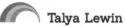
My Basic Meal – Healthy Speedy Sushi

During the summer I eat this, with variations, almost every day.

Dishes, for each person:

- A big bowl

- Chopsticks (so you eat more slowly, but if that doesn't work for you, use a knife and fork)

Ingredients:

- A large, delicious, colorful, fresh salad (refer to my rainbow salad at the end of this chapter)

- Place on top of the salad: 1/2 cup of cooked unflavored grains, either warm or cold (vary with quinoa, millet, brown rice, kasha or sometimes no grain at all. Refer to Step 15, Cooking Whole Grains, on page 203).

- A few tablespoons of whole tahini – sesame paste (refer to tahini at the end of this chapter)

- Choose from and vary: steamed vegetables, legumes, baked sweet potato, organic free-range hard-boiled egg, baked salmon, olives, avocado, sardines (in olive oil).

- A few sheets of nori seaweed (on the side). If possible, I recommend getting the raw organic kind.

Are You Ready to Eat?

So, you have your bowl, filled with a BIG yummy salad. On top you have some olives, a grain, tahini (on top or to the side) and other foodstuffs you choose and rotate. Here comes a great trick which helps crowd out bread: we all love our sandwiches. There is nothing wrong with having healthy bread every now and then, but many of us seem to eat too much bread. So, this little trick helps us eat less.

Ready?

Fold the nori sheet into fourths and tear into four smaller squares. Take one square and place a bit of salad + grain + tahini + anything else in the middle (you can also add a little soy sauce), fold over and eat.

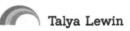
I call this **sushi to-go!** Great little delicious healthy sandwiches. So instead of eating so much bread, crowd it out by making nori sandwiches. I personally still eat bread but I honestly make these rolls with many of my meals. Beware – it is "addictive." And kids love it, too.

 Tip:

You can also make "rolls" with lettuce leaves, cabbage or any other big leaf.

Even if you don't like the nori leaves or the tahini, it's OK. The secret is making the salad large and very rich and placing other foods in smaller portions on top or on the side and eating sloooowly. Enjoy each and every bite. Remember to give your chopsticks a chance.

Get going and try it. Let me know how it goes.

 Nori Tip:

To keep the nori fresh, freeze it in a Ziploc bag.

In the winter or on colder days you can still have this meal but then I recommend making the salad a bit smaller and having lots of steamed or baked warm veggies, stews and other warm foods on top or mixed in. Most of us do better with cooked warm foods during autumn and winter.

Nomi and Tal's Healthy Roll

This is an invention of my sister Nomi and Tal, who was her business partner. Since they are both artists they naturally redesigned my original Sushi To Go, to become the Lufi.

Lafa is a thin sandwich pita roll, in Hebrew, and the Lufi is a combination of the lafa and sushi.

Make a lafa with a nori sheet. Place the whole nori sheet on a board or plate. Place grains, salad, sliced steamed veggies, sprouts, avocado, whatever you have, fold up the bottom, fold in one side and roll, so everything won't fall out the bottom, and roll (it should look like a big uncut sushi roll). Dunk into some olive oil, tahini or soy sauce and take a bite (may be rolled ahead of time or at the table by each person).

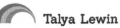

Whole Grains – Superlife's Healthy Habit Program

> Remember to add in different kinds of greens and raw vegetables gradually. Let your system slowly adjust to digesting the many fresh veggies and especially greens. If you aren't accustomed to eating many leafy greens, you might at first feel bloated; decrease the amount of greens and have a smaller salad. Gradually, step by step, enlarge the salad and greens until you find what works best for you.

My Basic Salad or My Rainbow Salad

Let the artist within you express itself and paint a salad, using as many colors as possible! Remember, each pigment has different healing properties. Create your salad, "painting" a colorful work of art.

Put a big pot in the sink and fill it with water and all the veggies you chose. Dry the LEAFY GREENS in the lettuce dryer, on a towel or just give them a good shake (the salad is so much tastier when the leaves are dry). Into a big salad bowl tear the lettuce by hand and chop up lots of other greens. Slice the other veggies. Here are a few suggestions:

- Lettuce varieties add many shades of green.

- Parsley/ coriander/ dill/ basil/ celery/ beet greens – these LEAFY GREENS provide iron and calcium in colors of deep dark green.

- Carrots for the orange – I love using a peeler to create long strips by peeling down the entire length of the carrot. Slice remaining core. I also love grating the carrots right into the salad for a natural sweet flavor.

- Fresh zucchini. Using a peeler, create long strips by peeling down the entire length of the zucchini. This gives a great texture.

- Tomatoes and red peppers for the wonderful joyful reds.

- Purple cabbage for a dark deep purple, cut into strips, full of healing antioxidants.

- Freshly grated ginger for an exciting change (best in the winter, to warm you up).

- And throw on lots of sprouts! This provides more shades of green (in the winter I would steam the sprouts a bit or leave them out, since they might be too cooling).

The Dressing

My favorite dressing, made by pouring and shaking right onto the salad (skip any ingredients that aren't to your taste):

Ingredients:

- Turmeric (amazing antioxidant), cumin (great for digestion), cinnamon (great for balancing sugar levels) – shake on generously.

- A little cayenne (a great superfood if you like some heat)

- Ground flax seeds (great source of omega 3 fatty acids and aid in bowel movement) – in the spice grinder, freshly grind about 1-2 tablespoons just before eating, as the pre-ground kind from health food stores loses most of its nutrients after a few hours.

- Pumpkin seeds (great source of omega 3 fatty acids)

- Olive oil, organic soy sauce – I just pour

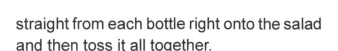
> straight from each bottle right onto the salad and then toss it all together.
>
> - A squirt of lemon (I love adding lemon to everything. There is something about it that upgrades everything. I also have a lemon tree in the garden, so it is very convenient.)

Other dressing options:

Olive oil + freshly squeezed lemon juice + Himalayan sea salt

Olive oil + balsamic vinegar + freshly ground flax seeds

Freshly squeezed lemon juice + tahini paste + soy sauce + sesame oil (add a bit of water and mix into a sauce)

Try adding other raw or steamed vegetables, seeds, nuts, seaweeds and superfoods (goji berries, hulled hemp seeds or cacao nibs taste great).

Mix it all together, making sure the flavor is delicious.

Lunch and Making a Rainbow Salad – Superlife's Healthy Habit Program

Tahini

A must at each meal – the best paste ever. Great on every food, instead of mayo. Try to find raw, organic, unshelled and sprouted – it's a wonderful source of protein, calcium and healthy fats. I like eating it in its natural state or making a spread. This spread can be refrigerated for a few days (I always have some ready in a glass jar) and is great on bread, grains, salad or cooked vegetables.

Ingredients – for 5 servings:

- 1/2 cup whole grain sesame paste

- 1/2 cup lemon juice (for a less sour taste, substitute some of the lemon juice with water or use mandarin juice for a sweet tahini)

»

- A lot of chopped greens (parsley, coriander, mint, basil or dill is delicious in the sweet tahini spread)

Directions:

1. In a bowl, hand-mix the sesame paste with the juice to form a smooth paste (you may add more juice or paste to vary the consistency).

2. Add chopped greens.

Healthy Oils – Superlife's Healthy Habit Program

Healthy Salts – Superlife's Healthy Habit Program

Step
9

What resonated with you? What are you going to try? Which leafy greens are you going to start with? When will you buy them? What will you make? Will you try rolling them in nori seaweed or any other leaf?

Go ahead – if you haven't jumped yet, it is time to – jump!

Remember: Patience and persistence is the name of the game.

My Basic Winter Meal
Simple, Delicious & Healthy

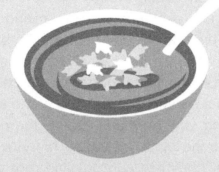

*Eat like a king in the morning,
a prince at noon, and a peasant at dinner.*

Maimonides – Rambam

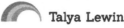

Continuing the theme of Step 10's quotation, what about, "Eat mostly green in spring, colors in summer and lots of orange in the fall and winter…"?

By now you know – I love salads! But I also used to freeze in the winter! Even during a mild "winter," I only defrosted when spring came around. It took me a while to realize there was a connection. I had never even considered that eating cold salads during wintertime was contributing to my shivers. But it actually makes sense. Today almost all fruits and vegetables are available all year round, and most of us don't even know what is really in season. But if you think about it, there is a reason certain foods grow at certain times of the year. Nature is brilliant, and there is a reason greens grow in the spring (they are cleansing, and spring is exactly the right time to cleanse after the winter), a variety of fruits grow in the summertime (they are cooling) and root vegetables, nuts and oily foods like avocados grow in wintertime (they are grounding and warming). The more we eat seasonally, the more balanced we will feel.

I solved the breakfast meal with the super morning porridge. And yet, when winter comes along, it sometimes is still hard for me to make the shift away from my delicious big salads at lunch to the more warming foods like soups and stews.

I don't spend much time in the kitchen. Here are two of the quickest, tastiest warming meals ever.

My Super Soup

I use whatever I have in the fridge but here is my basic recipe. It is really easy in a pressure cooker but can also be made in a large pot.

Ingredients – for 5 servings:

Group 1

Scrub and cut coarsely into big chunks (no need to peel – saves on time and preserves more of the nutrients):

- 2 medium onions (peeled)

- 1-2 tablespoons fresh ginger root (peeled and chopped)

- 2 sweet potatoes

- 2 potatoes

- 2 carrots

- 1 piece pumpkin or butternut squash »

- 1/4 teaspoon hot pepper (cayenne pepper is best)

- 1/3 teaspoon cinnamon

- 1/2 teaspoon turmeric

- 1 teaspoon cumin

- 3-4 cups water, or to just cover

Group 2

- 2 cloves garlic

- 1-2 tablespoons coconut oil

- 1-2 tablespoons soy sauce

- Freshly squeezed lemon juice

- Chopped fresh coriander for flavor and garnish

- You could also use lentils, beans or other legumes.

Directions:

1. Put all ingredients from Group 1 in the pressure cooker or large pot.

2. Add water just to cover, mix lightly and place lid on top.

In pressure cooker	In big pot
From the moment the pressure rises, cook for 2-3 minutes, then lower pressure immediately, cool and open.	Cut smaller pieces. Cook on medium heat for about 20 minutes until vegetables are tender. Or from the moment the water starts to boil, let simmer for 3-5 minutes, then cover and turn off heat, let sit covered for 30-40 minutes. The vegetables will cook by themselves.

3. Take half of the soup and put in a blender together with the garlic, coconut and soy ingredients from Group 2; blend till creamy.

4. Pour blended vegetables back into pot and mix together.

»

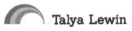

5. Or you can blend the whole amount into a creamy soup.

6. Adjust the flavor and add a bit more coconut oil or other condiments, to taste.

7. Serve with freshly squeezed lemon juice and chopped coriander.

Here is a video with a similar idea but a different recipe.

Whole Foods – Superlife's Healthy Habit Program

My Super Stew

This is very similar to the soup but still different and works with all types of legumes. I do recommend soaking legumes overnight, though the smaller ones like mung beans and lentils can be simply rinsed and drained. You are probably better off starting with lentils, since they are easy and quick to cook and digest. If you are using a pressure cooker, from the moment the pressure is reached, lentils should be cooked for 2-3 minutes only, otherwise they turn into a puree. When using beans, pressure cook them first until almost done, then lower the pressure and open the pot, adding the rest of the ingredients, and pressure cook again for 2-3 minutes, then lower pressure immediately and open.

Ingredients – for 5 servings:

Cut coarsely into big chunks, no need to peel (saves on time and preserves more of the nutrients):

- 1-2 tablespoons coconut oil or olive oil

- 1 cup lentils (soaked overnight or just rinsed)

- 2 medium onions (peeled)
- 1-2 tablespoons fresh ginger root (peeled and chopped)
- 4 cloves garlic
- 2 sweet potatoes
- 2 carrots
- 1/4 teaspoon cayenne pepper
- 1/2 teaspoon cinnamon
- 1 teaspoon turmeric
- 2 teaspoon cumin
- 2-3 tablespoon soy sauce
- 3 cups water, or just to cover
- Freshly squeezed lemon juice, chopped fresh coriander, for flavor and garnish

Directions:

1. Put lentils in pot with oil.

2. Add onion, ginger and garlic, and mix.

3. Add vegetables (place them on top without

mixing too much so it will also look nice once it is done – often I serve straight from my stainless steel pot).

4. Sprinkle spices on top and add soy.

5. Add water to just cover, and close pot.

In pressure cooker	In big pot
From the moment the pressure rises, cook for 2 minutes, then lower pressure immediately, cool and open.	Cook on medium heat for about 30 minutes. Add more water if needed.

6. Serve with freshly squeezed lemon juice and chopped coriander.

You could also add or substitute some of the veggies with:

- Leek (including green top)

- Piece of pumpkin or butternut squash

- Beets

- Small fennel

Since I have been living in a much colder climate for the last while (in Ireland), I have become more creative in the kitchen. It isn't that I spend more hours cooking – everything I cook is always very speedy and simple – but as far as my green smoothie and beautiful colorful green salads go, I realized they weren't going hand in hand with the Irish climate. I had to go a bit wild in the kitchen in order to keep them in my diet.

So here are a few more ideas:

Warm Up Your Salad

Put warm food right on top of the salad. Make the salad the base and put the warm food, whether it is whole grains, steamed or cooked vegetables or other warm dishes, straight on the salad.

Make a Soulad (Soup + Salad)

Throw lots of greens into your soup, or even throw the whole salad into the soup.

Use Warming Condiments

Certain foods are known to warm you up; like cinnamon, turmeric, cayenne, cumin, ginger. Add them to your salads, soups, smoothies and other dishes.

Smoothies

In colder weather I don't use ice in my green smoothie, and while in the summer I load up my smoothie with greens, in the winter I use fewer of them.

Step 10

So ... how are you doing so far?

What have you accomplished so far? What are you taking from this chapter?

Which recipe will you try: the Super Soup or Super Stew or the Salad?

Will you get yourself a pressure cooker?

Standing Up
To Your Word

*No. Try not. Do. Or do not.
There is no try.*

Yoda, Star Wars

I want to take a little break on our journey and remind you to really stand up to what you decided you would do.

You know how it is – you sometimes decide something but when the time comes to really do it there are a million reasons why not to. And then you start getting all confused: Should I do it? Should I go? Maybe I can cancel? I will do it tomorrow …

So when I make a decision about something and those voices come up, I acknowledge them, but then I just do what I decided I would do.

Why?

Because that is what I decided. That's it! That is the reason. It really simplifies things. I do it because I decided I would do it.

Then there is no chance to get confused. There is NO dilemma. I wake up in the morning and do yoga, because I decided I would.

And after I do it, I am always delighted.

My Tips For Cooking
Anyone Can Cook

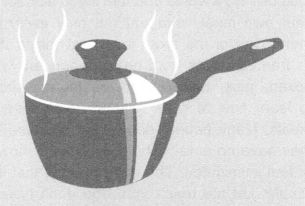

*Trust that still, small voice that says,
"This might work and I'll try it."*

Diane Mariechild

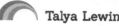

Do you cook?

How many times a week do you cook?

Honestly, when was the last time you cooked?

Today many people don't cook, but rather warm foods in the microwave, order takeaway or eat out. How much money would you save if you started cooking at home? How much healthier would your food be? How would you feel if you actually did cook your own meals and eat out only every now and then? One of the most important things that helps us free ourselves from being dependent on bought, boxed, junk, microwaved, restaurant, fastfood is to learn how to cook simple, quick, tasty, healthy meals. Many people don't cook because they feel they have no time. Others don't know how to cook or feel intimidated. The good news is that it is really simple. Let me teach you. You don't have to be a great chef in order to cook your own and your own family's meals. I'm not talking gourmet – that is OK once in a while – I'm talking simple, delicious and wholesome. When you cook your own food you know exactly what ingredients you used, you are in control of it being clean and fresh. And you can put your own energy and love ("Vitamin L," a forgotten vitamin) into the food, which is so very important.

Here are a few overall tips:

Use a Timer

Even if a dish takes 40 minutes to cook, you certainly don't have to be watching over it the whole time. You can turn on the timer and use the time to do other stuff. I put a pot of quinoa on the stove, turn on the timer for 20 minutes, and when it rings, turn it off. It is as simple as that.

Simplify the Recipes

Cook gourmet once in a while. I cook reallllly simply – and it's delicious. There are many recipes to make, even if you don't have some of the ingredients. If you don't have coriander, garlic, cinnamon, don't let that stop you from making a recipe you are looking at. But also, simplify the recipe.

Cook Once – Eat Twice or Three Times

Make big enough amounts so you have leftovers.

A. Grain example

- Cook a plain grain and make "My Basic Summer Lunch Meal" on page 127.

- For the next meal, stir fry the leftover grain with vegetables, ginger, garlic and soy sauce.

- Take the leftover stir fry to work the next day.

B. Vegetable example

Steam lots of different vegetables and root vegetables and eat them with a dressing of olive oil and soy sauce with a bunch of cut greens, a grain and some tahini.

For the next meal, mix the leftover vegetables into a salad and make "My Basic Summer Lunch Meal" on page 127.

For dinner rewarm the veggies, throw them into the blender with some warm water and condiments and make "My Super Soup" from "My Basic Winter Meal" on page 149.

C. Fish example

- Bake a whole salmon with root vegetables and eat them with a salad.

- For the next meal, make "My Basic Summer Lunch Meal."

- Take leftovers to work the next day or make a salmon sandwich with the leftover fish.

My favorite condiments – I use them in almost everything:

Cinnamon: sweet taste, great for digestion and for balancing blood sugar levels

Cumin: acts against gas and aids digestion

Turmeric: anti-inflammatory, one of the best antioxidants, lowers cholesterol, aids digestion, counteracts menstrual pains and more

Ginger: warming, acts against gas and aids digestion

Pink Himalayan salt: healthy salt, loaded with minerals, instead of the refined, white bleached stuff

Big Pot in Sink

When you start cooking, place a big pot in the sink, fill with water and throw all the greens in – it is so much easier to wash them this way. Drain the pot (you can use the water to water the plants), refill and rinse again, then move the greens to a towel or a lettuce dryer. Do the same with all the other veggies. Somehow it makes it easier and saves on water, too. I also use the lettuce dryer to refrigerate washed and unused greens and vegetables.

Food for Thought: There is nothing wrong with eating out. I love going out, especially for sushi. But I was a waitress for many years, and so I know that sometimes what you see "onstage" isn't what is happening "backstage."

Another very important and forgotten vitamin is "Vitamin H" – Homemade Food. The same salad made at home or in a restaurant – where they are making 10 other dishes all at the same time and have to get the food out quickly – has totally different energy and nutrients. The same food cooked at home with your own energy may be much more nourishing.

Step
11

Refer to the previous or following steps on how
to cook easy, tasty, digestible leafy greens,
whole grains, legumes, sprouts, root vegetables.
Choose one recipe and make it.

Remember: Cooking is like any other
art. It takes time to master. PLEASE don't be
hard on yourself, and don't give up if the first,
second or third time, something doesn't turn out
the way you planned. It is OK to make mistakes.
I promise you that the more you do it, the easier
it will become and the better you will be at it. Like
anything else you do.

Snacking
The Healthy Way

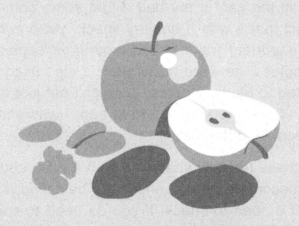

*It is always the simple things
that change our lives.*

Donald Miller

I used to be a "nosher" (a *snacker* in Yiddish), sweets mostly. In high school I constantly had chewing gum in my mouth and sometimes I would even fall asleep with it. Ever since I can remember, I recall eating apples, and a lot of them! I made a rough calculation and I estimate I ate at least 27,000 apples. I ate the whole apple, including the seeds, leaving only the stem which you could find all over the house, in my bags, in the car, in my bed. I find some comfort in the fact that it was a healthy snack, yet one of the most important fruits to eat organic is apples and the apples I ate were not organic. I also used to be addicted to Medjool dates. I couldn't eat just one or two – I'd go through the whole bag. I was addicted to chocolate, too.

Over these last few years, as both my life and food have become healthier and more balanced, I have less of a need to snack. If you do need to snack, I recommend asking yourself:

1. Am I eating meals?

2. Am I eating my meals with awareness? Am I chewing?

3. Do I have enough food during meals? Am I satisfied?

4. What is my stress level? Am I overworked? Overstressed?

5. Do I sleep enough? Am I tired?

6. Do I drink too much coffee?

7. Am I happy in my relationships?

8. Am I satisfied with my career?

9. Do I do enough physical activity? Do I move my body?

10. Do I have an activity that is meaningful to me beyond the physical world?

💡 Tips to deal with snacking:

1. If you find yourself eating too much, thinking of food and snacking, please consider the issues above. We will address them in Step 17 "Focus on Your Life Being Healthy and Emotional Eating" on page 225.

2. Most important – clear the house of all those tempting, toxic, unhealthy foods, like cakes and cookies, chips, candies, unhealthy chocolate and ice cream … and upgrade them to healthier options. You can't eat the whole ice cream carton with a teaspoon at midnight if it isn't in the fridge,

can you? Please be aware that we often buy foods "for the kids," "for my husband/ wife," "for the guests," but honestly, who is the one who ends up eating most of it? Good Question!

Do yourself and your loved ones a favor: don't have any of that in the house.

> If you absolutely need to have a little something unhealthy, have a small portion when you are out, but don't let any of it cross the entrance door.

Here is a list of healthy snacks to have at home, for you, for the kids, for your husband/ wife, for the guests …

Fruit

Apples, pears, mango, papaya, banana, watermelon, melon, grapes, citrus. Bananas are very sweet, so don't overdo it. You can also eat fruit with a few nuts to stabilize blood sugar levels.

Dried Fruit

Dates, raisins, apricots, figs, prunes. I recommend eating them together with some nuts or cacao nibs to stabilize blood sugar levels, since they too are very high in sugar.

Nuts

Almonds, walnuts, pistachios, macadamia, pecans, cashews, hazelnuts, brazil nuts. It is easy to overdo it with nuts, especially if you eat straight out of the package while doing something else, so put some in a little dish and eat with awareness. I also recommend eating unsalted, unroasted nuts, since the roasting at a high temperature destroys most the delicate nut fats and creates free radicals. Moreover, the oils and salt that are used in the commercial roasting of nuts aren't the healthy kinds. If you love roasted nuts, you could roast your own at a lower temperature.

I personally stay away from peanuts. Peanuts are often contaminated with a toxin called aflatoxin, which are said to be one of the highest carcinogens there are (this information is from The China Study, the most comprehensive study of nutrition ever conducted).

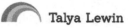

Breads

Rye bread, sprouted bread, spelt bread, gluten free breads. I eat them with tahini and vegetables; with avocado, a sliced tomato and olive oil; or with coconut oil, tahini and a healthy sweetener (like honey, maple syrup or silan) and some cacao nibs.

Superfoods

Raw cacao beans, goji berries.

Real Dark Chocolate

Choose at least 70% cacao.

Sugar Cravings – Superlife's Healthy Habit Program

Here Are a Few Of My Favorite Daily Snacks

Medjool Dates with Tahini, Coconut Oil and Cacao Nibs

This is the easiest and tastiest dessert ever invented!! It is great as a little energy booster during the day. It includes two of my favorite foods: cacao and dates. You can't go wrong.

Ingredients – for 1 serving:

- 2 large medjool dates
- Raw unhulled tahini
- Coconut oil
- Cacao nibs

Directions:

1. Open the dates and discard the pit.
2. Inside each half, spread tahini and some coconut oil and sprinkle with cacao nibs.

And voila! Done! This truly is divine.

You can easily have this at work. All you need to do is keep a stock of dates, tahini, coconut oil and cacao nibs there.

The dates have a great natural sweetness, and the coconut oil is a very healthy oil. I always recommend eating dried fruit with a healthy oil so your blood sugar doesn't go spiking. And cacao gives a great crunch together with lots of antioxidants, minerals and a light energy boost. No wonder cacao is named Theobroma Cacao – Food of the Gods.

You can make it with only tahini, or with only coconut oil, and also add some goji berries or walnuts.

Toast with Coconut Oil, Tahini, Silan and Cacao Nibs

Here is another delicious quick snack. Instead of using dates, you can spread the mix on toast or spelt bread. When I spread it on toast, I put a generous amount of coconut oil first, since it melts right in, then the tahini and silan on top and sprinkle with cacao nibs.

My Amazing CHOCOLATE RECIPE

> *Put 'eat chocolate' at the top of your list of things to do today. That way, at least you'll get one thing done.*
>
> The Rules of Chocolate

My father was originally from Belgium, and so while I was growing up, we often had Leonidas or Godiva chocolates in the house. They weren't as widely known or available as today, and to have them was a real treat (actually, it still is).

After dinner we would have the ceremony of going to the fridge and bringing out the golden box with the fancy dainty papers. My sister and I would carefully open the box and examine each praline, choosing "the right one" to eat at that moment.

We would nibble it very slowly, treating it as though it were something precious, relishing each bite. Without paying much attention, my father would just take a chocolate and quickly pop the whole thing into his mouth, and we would howl every time, not understanding his haste. He would laugh, while chewing and swallowing it soon after.

Growing up that way, I have always LOVED chocolate. So finding out that chocolate can be healthy was a very exciting discovery for me. I learned how to make it when I was studying nutrition. I have been making and eating my own homemade version of delicious chocolate for quite a while and I love sharing it with the whole world. Because we all love chocolate – research shows that chocolate is the food women crave most – you are better off eating the real thing. Beware! Once you taste this chocolate, you'll be hooked forever. It is free of refined sugar, gluten, cholesterol, milk products, soy, flour and preservatives, all ingredients that are in many of the industrial chocolate products.

Make Your Own Organic Raw Chocolate

Ingredients:

- 1/2 cup of coconut oil
- 1/4 cup of ground cacao beans (or nibs)
- 1 cup of cacao powder (or 1.5 cups of powder – no beans)
- 1/3 cup of maple syrup

»

Directions:

1. Line a low pan with parchment paper.

2. Use cacao nibs or grind cacao beans in coffee grinder (or in food processor or strong blender).

3. In a bowl combine cacao powder and cacao nibs.

4. Melt oil in pot over water on very low flame, but don't overheat.

5. Add maple syrup to the oil and mix.

6. Add the cacao nibs and cacao powder and mix well.

7. Add one of the following flavors, mix and place in pan, refrigerate.

Flavors:

<u>Cayenne</u> – a carrier of the benefits of cacao, straight to the cells. Expands the capillaries allowing the cacao to reach the cells more easily.

<u>Cinnamon</u> – stabilizes blood sugar.

<u>Mint</u> – the only green leafy food that really works well with cacao. Contains high levels of calcium, which works really well with the magnesium in cacao (since you need magnesium to absorb calcium).

<u>Orange Zest</u> – freshly grated

<u>Tahini</u> – pour straight on top of chocolate in pan and use a fork to swirl a beautiful design.

Or try these flavors: goji or other berries, dried fruits, nuts, raisins, coconut shreds, bee pollen, carob, maca (works great with cacao), vanilla.

Tip:

If you would like the chocolate bar to stay hard out of the fridge, you can substitute cacao butter for the coconut oil. But if you do, make sure it is organic cacao butter and not too processed. When using coconut oil you will have to keep the chocolate refrigerated, since coconut oil melts quite quickly.

Check out the recipe section on page 275 at the end of the book for other healthy sweets.

Remember: When you do have a snack, no matter what it is (even if it is ice cream), eat it with awareness.

This is how to snack with full awareness:

1. Ask yourself if you are bored, upset or stressed and see if you can find a different solution to "the situation" besides eating, like going out for a walk, practicing yoga, reading, meeting a friend, getting a hug, giving a hug, going to a movie, or dancing. Do something you love, meet someone you love and notice how you suddenly don't have as much of a desire to eat.

2. If you do decide to eat something, put it on a plate.

3. Sit down.

4. Do nothing else besides eating – eat with full awareness.

5. Enjoy it. No guilt allowed.

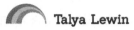

What do you think about clearing your kitchen of all the tempting, toxic, unhealthy foods and upgrading them? What healthy snacks can you get instead? When are you going to do it? What flavor will you put in your homemade chocolate?

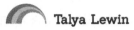 **Remember:** Life is to be enjoyed. If it isn't fun – it isn't worth it.

How to Eat
Teachings of My 95-Year-Old Grandmother

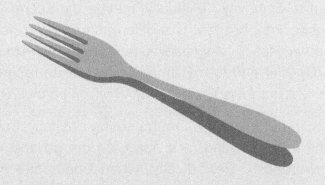

I have made it a rule to give every tooth of mine a chance, and when I eat, to chew every bite thirty-two times. To this rule I owe much of my success in life.

William Gladstone

The How Is Often More Important Than the What

My grandmother passed away at the age of 95 and 4 months. Bless her! I think one of her most valuable secrets (besides drinking coffee and enjoying chocolate) is that she was a slow eater. When I say slow, I mean **REALLY** s-l-o-w! When we were well into our main course, she was still sipping her soup. Every bite was delivered to the mouth in slow motion and chewed, thoroughly. Could this have been her secret to longevity? (Actually, maybe the secret was the chocolate, but that is a different subject. Refer to Cacao in Step 7 "Upgrade Yourself With Superfoods" on page 94 and to my amazing chocolate recipe in Step 12 "Snacking The Healthy Way" on page 178.)

I must admit that even though eating healthily, I used to find myself eating in a hurry, on the go and with no awareness. Periodically, when under stress or unhappy, I was swallowing without really chewing. Actually eating with awareness and really chewing is a more difficult task than it seems.

Today, eating doesn't seem to be considered an action on its own. When I ask my clients why they don't sit and eat but rather multi-task while eating, most reply that it is boring or a waste of time. Isn't that weird? So many of us are so preoccupied with our food; we feel we love eating, but then when we eat we actually do something else: read a book or the newspaper, work at the computer, watch TV, drive, walk, eat on the go. You will rarely see someone just sit and eat. I want you to consider that eating is an action on its own, just like showering or brushing your teeth.

Here comes your next best tip ever!!! I think it actually is one of the hardest, but most important of all.

When you eat, you only eat. You do nothing else. Whether it is a meal, a snack or just a nibble, you do it with full awareness. Put the food on a plate and sit down at the table. No multi-tasking! I promise you, this is life-transforming. Do not allow yourself to eat while reading or doing anything else. If you do, you will eat much more than you need and you will miss out on the whole experience, finding yourself unsatisfied, eating all day long, going back and forth to the fridge.

Please consider these points.

1. What Are We Absorbing?

When we eat, our body is very open. We don't only absorb the nutrients from the food, we absorb everything that is around us. Imagine what kind of energy we are absorbing if we eat in a calm environment (like out in nature) versus eating in a noisy restaurant, driving on the highway. What energy are we taking in, listening to the morning news while having our breakfast? Try cherishing the meal, finding a calm, pleasant place to eat and absorb the nutrition, whether it is in the form of phytonutrients or environmental nutrients.

2. No Multi-Tasking at Mealtimes

Our brains are capable of concentrating on only one action at a time. In our western world we are used to multi-tasking, but if while we are eating, we are watching TV, working at the computer or reading, our brain is focused on that other action. We aren't really focused on eating, we don't really chew and the food doesn't get digested properly (resulting in gas, stomach aches and other problems). We also don't really know we have eaten, so we eat more than we need.

3. Which Nervous System Should Be Activated?

The nervous system that is responsible for digestion is the parasympathetic one, the same one that controls the practices of meditation, yoga and relaxation. But when we are eating on the go, the nervous system that is in charge is the sympathetic one – the one that activates the "fight or flight" response when we actually want to be in "rest and digest" mode. Before eating take a few deep breaths, relax, feel your stomach, your pelvis and your feet, ground yourself and let the proper nervous system come into action.

4. Digestion Begins in the Mouth

The digestion of complex carbohydrates begins in the mouth with the enzyme amalyze, which breaks them down into simple sugars and makes fats, minerals and proteins capable of maximum absorption. It makes sense that our food should be chewed well before swallowing.

Remember: The stomach doesn't have any teeth.

Food for Thought: Is there a chance that peace on earth can begin by all of us chewing? Each person will chew and slowly relax. Then the family will chew and relax. Then the street, the neighborhood, the city, the country ... everyone will calm down and be happy, and it will all begin by chewing the food in our mouths. Chewing ... relaxing ... how simple is that?!

Steps For Slow and Aware Daily Eating

Try to be in a good mood, if you aren't you will often eat much more than you need to, and without awareness. So check your mood; if you are low see if there is any way you can be more positive.

1. Find a quiet, comfortable place to eat.

2. Make a plate – don't be stingy and don't overdo it. Make a plate you feel comfortable with.

3. Look at the food before you begin eating – appreciate all that abundance. Think of the process the food went through before it got to your plate. Many of the foods were originally seeds that were planted. See if you can see Nature in your food.

4. Take a deep breath – or a few deep breaths. Stimulate your parasympathetic nervous system. Feel your center.

5. Use chopsticks, or a small spoon or fork; this helps to slow down and take smaller bites, instead of using the fork like a tractor shovel.

6. Between bites put down the cutlery.

7. Count your chews. How many chews for each mouthful? Did your food turn to a more liquid form before swallowing or are you barely chewing?

8. Put your awareness in your mouth, in the food that is in your mouth and not on the next bite. It really helps to even close your eyes while chewing.

9. Notice the difference between eating like this and eating while barely chewing, on the go. Notice if you feel more satisfied, lighter, if your digestion is better. You could fill in "Your Personal Lab Test" Chart from Step 8 on page 124 for other meals besides breakfast.

This isn't easy – it demands practice. But it is revolutionary. It is life-transforming.

Don't believe me; you have to try it out for yourself. Instead of putting the emphasis on calories and counting your food, put it on chewing your food. We have an opportunity to practice yoga, meditation, observation, relaxation, and slowing down a few times a day, every time we eat. Make eating the practice of eating. Make "how you eat" your daily practice.

> *He who prolongs the time at the table –*
> *prolongs his life.*
>
> The Rambam

Step
13

I am going to be strict with this step, because I truly feel it is one of the most important of all, if not THE most important. From now on, when you eat – you only eat. You do nothing else! No reading, no watching TV, no working on the computer, no eating in the car ... Whether it is a meal, a snack or just a nibble, you sit and eat with full awareness. Make a conscious decision to eat with awareness, and I promise you will have a totally different eating experience. When you sit at the table, maybe play some relaxing music, thank the food and your life, and then take a bite and really chew. A day of aware eating and chewing is a totally different day than one of hasty eating and swallowing with no presence.

Remember: This step is one of the hardest, and it really takes practice and persistence, trying over and over and over again. It is probably a lifelong job. You will find yourself eating slowly and losing it every time. When that happens bring the awareness back to your mouth, to the taste, to the chewing, to your breath. Even if you only are aware for a few minutes during each meal, that is fine. Your ability to eat with awareness will grow the more you pay attention to it.

Step

14

Healthy On The Go
The Lunch Box

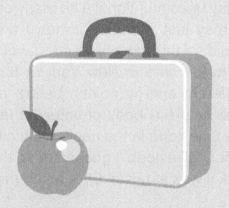

Anything is possible…

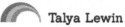

Traveling or Taking Food to Work

Many times when we are traveling or on the go, it is hard to eat healthily. However it really is very easy to put together a delicious nourishing lunch box. During the years I studied nutrition in New York, I was more in the air than on the ground. The unique curriculum allowed me to live in Israel, study long-distance through the net and phone calls and fly to New York about once a month. Those years of my life were very unconventional (like many other things I do) and they just "flew" by. When I boarded the plane I would go through my little ritual of tuning my meridians to the time in New York (a technique of tapping different energy points, before and during the flight to help the body counter jet lag and set itself to the time zone in the destination city). Before takeoff I often fell asleep, I guess due to the fact that in New York it was almost 4:00 A.M. Or maybe I was just tired ...

I remember one flight quite vividly. Forty minutes after takeoff I felt someone touching my arm. I opened my eyes, and the stewardess was holding a tray that said VEG on it.

"Would you like to eat?" she asked.

Instead I asked myself, "Did she have to wake me?"

There was an empty seat between me and the other passenger, an elderly man in his late 70s, and I opened the table to that seat and said, half asleep, "Please put it here." They always bring the vegetarian (which I ordered) and the kosher meals before serving everyone else, so my VEG meal sat between me and the elderly man – Alex, who later told me his whole life story. In the meantime I fell fast asleep again. The next time I opened my eyes, Alex had "MY" vegetarian meal on his table and was in the midst of opening the warm tofu dish. Instinctively I said, "That's mine!" but immediately, remembering that I actually brought my own food, added, "It's OK! I have my own."

All I needed from the airplane meal tray was the cutlery. So Alex was eating my vegetarian meal, and from my own bag I took out my healthy flight meal. Sushi to go!

I likely seemed a little weird to the people sitting near me on the flight, but deep down I think they would have paid to switch to my healthy meal. It always encouraged a conversation about health and food, and I even got a few clients on board.

Here Is My Lunch Box

You can mix your lunch all together in one box (or flask), or put it in separate little boxes. Don't stay attached to this example; rather get inspired to do your own – actually, anything can work.

1. A plastic box (one from high-quality plastic that can be reused) filled with a colorful salad, made from a variety of many green leaves and herbs, vegetables, and spices. On top I place a little tightly tied plastic bag, containing olive oil and soy sauce (the dressing).

2. A little plastic box with cooked whole grain rice (or quinoa, kasha, millet or any other whole grain) with homemade tahini sauce poured on top.

3. A little plastic box with beans (any kind, or peas).

4. A Ziploc bag with a few sheets of nori seaweed.

When I am ready to eat I make a little hole in the bag and squirt the dressing onto the salad, close the box and shake it around, so the dressing coats all. I tear the nori sheets into four smaller squares and place a bit of rice, beans and salad in the middle of each piece, fold and eat. If it is a long flight, I always order the vegetarian meal, but at least I am set with my healthy meal for the beginning.

If I can't or have no time to prepare this meal, I will go to a restaurant that has a good salad bar and make myself a box for the way or make a few sandwiches.

I honestly believe that had I been eating the airplane

food (industrial, canned, processed, full of chemicals, preservatives, herbicides, salt, sugar, white flour ...), I wouldn't have made it to the end of the school year.

> Intentionally cook more food for dinner than you need, so you have some for your lunch box for the next day.

Other good treats I take with me when I'm moving around, eat "as-is" or add to dishes:

1. Dried fruit (dates, goji berries, mulberries) and nuts (almonds, brazil, walnuts, cashews)

2. Superfoods: cacao nibs, goji berries, maca, chia, hemp seeds, spirulina (can be added to bought shakes, salads, porridge, yogurt)

3. Apples or any other sturdy fruit

4. Carrots, cucumbers or celery

5. Organic dark chocolate (at least 70% cacao)

6. Dates, tahini and cacao nibs (of course!)

7. Oats to make a porridge (if you can't cook them, you may also soak them overnight and just add

nuts, goji berries, a sliced banana and superfoods to the raw soak)

8. Tahini and honey to spread on bread or use as a sauce

In Restaurants

As mentioned earlier there are two very important vitamins that are lacking in most restaurant/ bought food: Vitamin H and Vitamin L.

That said, I also enjoy eating out where – though it is more difficult to control the amount of salt, sugar, unhealthy fats and other ingredients that go into the food – we can always make healthy choices.

1. **Salad**. I often look for the salad section on the menu first and find a big salad. If there are any ingredients I don't want I ask to leave them out or serve them on the side. Sometimes I ask for substitutes. I ask for an olive oil-based dressing (if it's not the one offered) and have no problem having them put it right on the salad. It is usually much tastier all mixed in, and if it is good olive oil, that is fine.

2. **Adding**. I add a dish from the starter menu and ask to have it served at the same time as the

salad. It isn't as big as the main course dish but will do fine with the big salad.

- Steamed/ baked/ cooked vegetables (with the sauce on the side, since many times it is a base of cream or butter).

- Fish

- Legumes

- Whole grain bread or grains. Many restaurants nowadays have quinoa or brown rice. In some restaurants you can even order sushi made with brown rice.

3. **Warm dishes**. Other times I will order a soup (not made with cream or milk) or a main course dish with a smaller salad. If the main course dish has a salad and French fries or a different side dish I don't want I ask for double salad or a substitution.

4. **My 20 percent.** If you feel you do want something "unhealthy" (whether it is pizza, pasta, falafel...), always, always, always have the best quality and add a salad. Make sure to leave the guilt at home. No point eating something and feeling guilty. We don't have to be fanatic about it. Remember, 80 percent of the time we eat healthy food, 20-30 percent of the time we "don't" – and that is perfect.

5. **Portions**. Sometimes the portions are really huge. Look around to see what people are eating or ask the waiter. Depending on how hungry I am and how big the portions are, many times the small portion works fine along with a big salad (though I always order the large salad).

6. **Sharing**. Often it is great to share with your eating companion. Share the main course or share the salad or do both. That way, both of you are in the same energy vibe. You won't be eating one order big enough for two, wanting to finish, not wanting to waste, going into automatic eating, leaving the table feeling stuffed.

We can always create the reality we want, and when we eat out we can ask to switch and change, so it works for us. We don't have to stay exactly with the menu.

What is the worst thing that can happen? They could say no, but most often restaurants willingly oblige.

Step
14

So ... how is the previous step, Step 13, going for you? I told you it was a hard one ... Now out of everything that was mentioned in this chapter, what is your next step?

Here are a few options:

Will you take a lunch box to work? If so, when?

Will you cook dinner and take the leftovers with you?

Will you take snacks with you? Which ones?

When eating out, what changes will you try to implement?

 Remember to take baby steps!

Cooking Whole Grains
How, What & Why

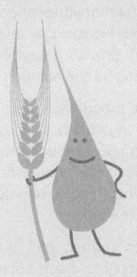

*The awareness of imbalance
is the first step in creating balance.*

Paul Pitchford

What Is a Whole Grain?

Think about it like this – white rice is naked, while whole grain brown rice has its clothes on. A processed grain is stripped of the bran (containing the fiber, B vitamins and trace minerals), the germ (containing B vitamins, vitamin E, trace minerals and enzymes) and is mostly a carbohydrate. When we eat a whole grain, the sugar (carbohydrates) goes into our blood slowly, keeping our blood sugar level stable (and our mood stable, too), providing sustainable high-quality energy, while giving us the nutrition nature created.

When we eat a processed grain (white rice and white flour, among others) it is deficient in all the nutrients, making us eat much more than we need since our body, designed to eat whole foods, doesn't understand this incomplete, unnatural, refined food and cries out for nutrition.

We feel hungrier sooner, our blood sugar levels spike up quickly only to crash soon after leaving us feeling "hungry" (we aren't – it is the sugar crash), irritable, low, tired, fat and eventually ill.

Epidemiological studies indicate that diets rich in whole grains are associated with lower risk of coronary heart disease and type 2 diabetes.

Here is a scenario of a normal day in a person's life:

The day begins with a cup of coffee with sugar and some processed food like a muffin, white bread or boxed cereal – sugar levels rise, we feel energetic.

We find ourselves a few hours later needing another boost of energy, so we go automatically for another cup of coffee with sugar, a cookie, a processed sweet, a carbonated drink loaded with sugar – sugar levels spike again.

At lunchtime we gulp down (in the car, in front of the computer, in a noisy restaurant) a pizza, pasta, bread, or white rice, all processed carbohydrates that keep us going for a few more hours until the big crash. (Imagine yourself going downhill on that big roller coaster.) Somewhere in the afternoon we have that three o'clock slump. We try to solve it with some more coffee, another carbonated drink or something sweet.

Isn't that what many of us go through all day, every day, for all our life? And every time sugar levels fall, so does our mood.

It doesn't have to be like this!

No wonder nowadays kids have early-onset diabetes – not too long ago it was a sickness affecting only those of 60 years and over. Now it is normal that kids will

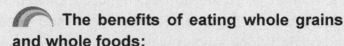

have diabetes type 2, a sickness that is closely linked to heart disease, stroke and other serious illnesses. The pancreas isn't supposed to be working around the clock, trying to stabilize our sugar level spikes due to eating so much sugary and processed foods.

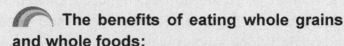 **The benefits of eating whole grains and whole foods:**

- Full of all the nutrients nature created

- Provides long lasting energy

- Keeps blood sugar levels stable

- Keeps moods stable

How to Cook Whole Grains

Many people complain that whole grains take too long to cook and aren't tasty.

 Tip:

Soak the grains overnight in a pot of water before cooking. In the morning discard the water and cook (you don't have to stand near the stove, but instead, use the timer). If you have no time to cook them, you can keep the pot of grains in the soaking water refrigerated for a few days.

Why Soak?

The soaking starts a process of germination, and the sprout starts coming alive, adding loads of nutrition. The sprouting process also neutralizes the phytic acid that is around grains. This acid stops grains from sprouting, otherwise everything would be sprouting all over the place, but it isn't healthy for us, since it prohibits the absorption of minerals.

My Basic Grain – Simplified

I often cook grains smply, not even adding salt, only water. Once the grain is cooked, I can play around with it. I also often cook the grains in the morning (using a timer) so when lunch comes around I have some food already prepared; otherwise I find myself going to bread or a quick fix.

Step 1: Soak and cook

- 1 cup of whole grain – soak overnight (or for eight hours) in water to cover.

- The next day, rinse grains, then bring to a boil in fresh water. If cooking oats, cook in their soaking water.

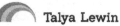

- Once it comes to a boil, put on the timer for 20 minutes. (Oats take 10 minutes.) Cook on a low flame.

Step 2: Eat

Refer to Step 9 "My Basic Summer Lunch Meal" on page 127.

- Mix it into a salad (refer to quinoa salad in recipe section).

- Pour olive oil and soy sauce on grains – so simple but so delicious.

- Stir fry with other vegetables. Refer to the recipe section.

Here are some of the basic whole grains I cook:

Grains/ 1 Cup	Soaking Time	Cook with	Cooking Time	Nutrition Info	Cooking Tips
Quinoa	I don't soak. Just rinse well.	2 cups water	20 min	Very healthy and high in protein Gluten-free	Mix white/red/black together.
Buckwheat (kasha) Actually a seed, but eaten as a grain	Overnight or for 8 hours	2 cups water	15 min	Very healthy and high in protein Gluten-free	Great to stir fry with shitake mushrooms, peas, garlic and soy sauce
Millet	Overnight or for 8 hours	2 cups water	20 min	Very healthy and high in protein Gluten-free	Doesn't have much flavor. Needs to have things added – try green leaves, nuts, sesame/olive oil.

Grains/ 1 Cup	Soaking Time	Cook with	Cooking Time	Nutrition Info	Cooking Tips
Oats	Overnight or for 8 hours – I cook them in the soaking water.	Water to cover	10 min	Has gluten, since is packaged in factories that have wheat	Great for breakfast. Check out my Superfood Porridge.
Whole grain rice	Overnight or for 8 hours	2 cups water	20 min	Gluten-free	Try different varieties: long, round, Thai/ red
Wheat	Overnight or for 8 hours	2-3 cups water	35-40 min	Has gluten	Great in stews and soups

You can try mixing a few whole grains together.

**Whole Grains – Superlife's
Healthy Habit Program**

Step
15

Which whole grain will you cook?

Even if you feel intimidated … even if you have that voice that says "I can't cook" or "It won't be tasty" or "I have no time" or "I like white rice," I say, "Live dangerously," as my mother always said to me. Take chances – life will catch you. So, which whole grain will you cook? When will you buy it? When will you cook it?

Legumes & Sprouting
Powerful Plant Proteins

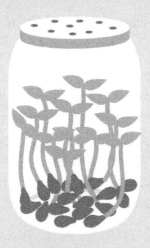

*Nothing will benefit human health
and increase the chances for
survival of life on Earth as much as
the evolution to a vegetarian diet.*

Albert Einstein

In this chapter we will focus on the legume family of beans and lentils, a great vegetarian source of protein, and on sprouting. Some people fear beans since they feel they are time-consuming to prepare, difficult to digest and not tasty. It would be a pity to miss out on this healthy family, so let me teach you all the little tricks that make a huge difference.

Let's Meet the Members of This Family

There are many different kinds of beans: adzuki (a Japanese dark red bean), chickpeas (high in protein and great for making homemade humus and Indian dishes or adding to other dishes), lima beans, peas, mung beans (a small bean that cooks very quickly) and many more. There are also different varieties of lentils: orange, yellow, green, brown – all delicious and quick to cook.

 Tip:

The smaller the bean, the quicker it cooks and the easier it is to digest.

What Is Healthy About Them?

They are an easy and animal-friendly way to add high-quality, plant-based protein to your diet. They are also high in magnesium (the most deficient mineral in peoples' diet today and very important for the heart), zinc, iron (magnesium, zinc and iron are great antidepressant minerals), B vitamins (important for the nervous system), fiber (besides moving the bowels, may aid in lowering cholesterol) and more.

> I recommend storing them – like grains – in glass jars, in a cool dark place or refrigerated, to keep fresh. An old bean will not soften easily in the cooking process, will be hard to digest and will be low on nutritional content. So keep them fresh!

It Is Very Important to Soak Your Beans (Just Like You Soak Your Grains)

In the same way as grains, the soaking starts a process of germination – the sprout starts coming alive, adding loads of nutrition and reducing cooking time. The soaking and sprouting process also neutralizes the phytic acid in beans, grains, nuts and seeds. As mentioned earlier in the book, this acid isn't healthy for us, since it prohibits the absorption of minerals (those amazing antidepressants, zinc,

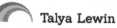

iron and magnesium, that we really want to absorb as much of as we can).

Lentils and small beans – like mung beans, peas and adzuki – need less soaking time, a minimum of eight hours up to 24 hours. Bigger beans like chickpeas and lima beans need longer to soak. Depending on the climate, they could soak up to three days. It is important to change the water every now and then.

After soaking, rinse and cook.

If you forgot or didn't presoak, you can put them in a pot, pour boiling water over them and bring them to a boil. Then turn off heat, cover and let sit for one hour.

 I often soak the small ones overnight, then rinse and cook them the following day.

A Few More Tips:

1. To soften beans, aid in digestion and add minerals add a small piece of kombu seaweed while cooking. Don't worry – even if you don't like seaweed, it will not influence the flavor.

2. To prevent gas, put beans in a large pot, cover with water, bring to a boil (uncovered) and skim off the foam (that is what actually creates the gas). Then cover and cook for remaining time.

3. About 10-15 minutes before the end of cooking, add some unrefined sea salt (don't add salt at the beginning since it contracts the beans, and they will not cook properly) and some organic apple cider vinegar (which softens the beans and aids in breaking down the chains of amino acids, therefore making them easier to digest and absorb).

4. Test for cooking: Beans are cooked when you squeeze them and the middle is soft and tender.

5. Other foods that aid in digesting beans are bay leaves, garlic, ginger, cinnamon, turmeric, cumin (powder or seeds), fennel seeds and coriander seeds. All great and tasty to add to the dishes.

6. Use a pressure cooker – saves on so much cooking time.

7. Many people add baking soda (sodium bicarbonate) to soften beans and vegetables. I would recommend avoiding that; while this will do the job of shortening cooking time and making them softer, baking soda may also interfere in the absorption of nutrients.

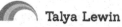

8. Make sure to chew your beans well (remember Step 13 "How To Eat").

Sprouting

If people commonly avoid cooking beans, they avoid sprouting them even more. It may seem like only "the health freaks" make their own sprouts, but it actually is very easy. YOU do nothing – Nature does all the work. And you get all the benefits.

Why Do I Call Sprouts "Super Sprouts"?

• Each seed, grain or bean has the potential of the whole plant dormant within. When we sprout them, the potential awakens: the bean absorbs water and multiplies in size, complex compounds breakdown into simpler forms and everything comes alive.

• The amount of starch and anti-nutrients decreases.

• The nutritional value and availability of different nutrients rise dramatically.

• The amount of vitamins can rise by 10 to 100 percent, sometimes even by 500 percent, especially the B group vitamins and other vitamins like vitamin E and beta carotene.

• Enzyme activity increases.

- Protein quality and quantity increases.

- The amount of fiber and antioxidants increases.

- Sugars become simple sugars – easy to digest.

If I've Inspired You, Here Is How Easy It Is to Sprout

1. I recommend starting off with the easy-to-sprout small legumes: mung beans, all lentils, adzuki or even grains like buckwheat, quinoa and wheat.

2. Rinse them well (make sure they are fresh, as old seeds will not sprout well).

3. Soak overnight (large ones might need longer, up to 48 hours).

4. Drain and rinse again. Place on a sprouting tray (there are many different kinds). You can also sprout in a jar that has holes in the top. After rinsing, you turn the jar upside down, and the water drains out (you can make your own or buy). I just use a strainer.

5. Place in a warm spot (but not in direct full sunlight where it could be too hot and dry them out).

6. Rinse two to four times a day. It is very important that the seeds stay moist and don't dry out, but

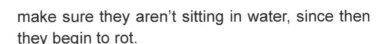

make sure they aren't sitting in water, since then they begin to rot.

7. After a few days they will have a little sprout and are ready to eat (in a warm climate mung beans, lentils and other small seeds can even sprout the same day).

8. When the sprout is about two centimeters long, place in a closed box and refrigerate.

9. Always rinse before eating to clean off any possible germs and bacteria.

10. You can sprout all types of beans, lentils, some nuts such as almonds, grains and grasses (like wheat grass).

11. It is easier to sprout in warm weather, so in winter the process will take longer.

How to Eat Sprouts

- Eat raw on salads, in sandwiches, sprinkle on warm dishes, as a beautiful garnish.

- Eat as a healthy snack (delicious with olive oil and a little soy sauce).

- Sauté with other veggies.

- Add to soups, stews or cooked grains.

Tip:

Sprouts have a cooling effect on the body, so it is better to eat them raw in warm weather. In the winter, if you are of a thinner body build or suffer from being cold, you can lightly steam or cook them.

> **Food For Thought:** Eat pulses for ecological reasons. Eat less meat, save our planet.

When I studied in New York City, we had a lecture about the animal food industry. Eric Schlosser, a journalist, author and one of the greatest food activists in the United States, gave us a very powerful slide lecture on the subject of the food industry, fast food, meat and the animals in our Western World. It was difficult to watch. There is so much that I can say on this close-to-my-heart subject. So many people feel they need to have meat for protein, but there really are other options, between the superfoods, the legumes or even eating smaller amounts of meat, fish, eggs and cheese. Everything has protein in it, even green leaves! We don't realize that meat and other animal food production requires huge amounts of energy, land, water and money. Cows for milk and meat produce tons and tons of feces. In the USA the waste is collected and stored in huge pools; it is full of antibiotics and hormones, polluting the soil and the water and discharging gas. One of the main reasons for global warming is actually the gas emitted from cows' feces. In America, one cattle factory alone produces in one day more feces waste than the cities Denver, Boston and St. Louis do together. There actually is more than enough land and money in the world to feed everyone, if we all ate less meat and more pulses. We must start to question our food choices and find alternatives, for us, for our children and for planet Earth.

Remember: Big changes begin with individuals, step by step!

Step
16

Was I able to inspire you to cook some legumes and to sprout?

What legume will you cook? What will you sprout? When will you buy them? When will you cook them? Try my Super Soup and Super Stew with different kinds of legumes.

Try my Basic Summer Meal with sprouts. Go ahead – jump, and the net will appear.

Focus On Your Life Being Healthy and Emotional Eating

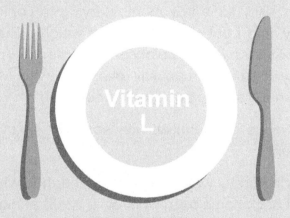

Vitamin L

Just as FOOD is needed for the BODY, LOVE is needed for the SOUL.

Osho

Eating healthily is just one part of the equation. In order to really be healthy and happy, we must have the courage to look at our lives.

All through my teenage years and up to my early 30s, I often went to food for the wrong reasons – when I was stressed, sad, worried, angry or bored. It wasn't apparent since I was always slim and most of the time in control of my food (except for when I went to University for a few months, trying to conform to society, and I put on quite a bit of weight). But even slim, I knew I wasn't balanced. Even if you turn to healthy food, you can still overdo it with Medjool dates, nuts, apples and gluten free bread.

Many of us are familiar with some or all of these situations.

- Eating pretty well all day long, and then when we get back home from work or at 22:00 at night, we have a "date" with the open fridge that leaves us feeling stuffed and guilty and saying to ourselves, "This will never happen again! Tomorrow, I am going on a diet."

- Nibbling all day long.

- Or just eating too much on a regular basis, leaving us carrying around our "heavy luggage."

I feel that many people **don't have an eating problem**, they have an **"unhappy life" problem**.

> If you want to solve your eating "disorder," to lose weight or to focus less on food in general, **make your life happy and you will not have an eating problem.**

It is true that it is easier said than done. But most people don't even want to go there, are scared of change and the unknown or rather feel it isn't possible, shut their eyes to the truth, bury their feelings, accept the status quo or pretend everything is OK and therefore continue carrying around their extra "heavy baggage."

For me there is no question. I want my life to be "light" and the best ever. After removing from my life everything that felt wrong, now:

I work in my passion (I don't even see it as work today).

I have a wonderful, loving relationship.

And I have lots of fun and enjoy living.

We all deserve that! We deserve to have an amazing life, an inspiring job and a loving, deep relationship.

Getting back to food, it will be really difficult and almost impossible to take control of your food if you aren't happy or living "your life." And many of us aren't living our lives. We are living our parents' dreams, society's pressures, our own pressure ... Though it may be a long process, it is totally possible to create the life of our dreams. Life is a l-o-n-g time. We better make it amazing! And then, we will really only go to food when we are hungry. (Of course a little snack every now and then is fine).

In today's world I feel people are compromising themselves in these main areas:

Work – either working too much or working in a job we don't like. Think about it: We spend most of our day at work. We put so much emphasis on what we wear, what we eat, where we live, whom we marry ... but most of the hours of the day and most of the days of the week we are at work. If we don't enjoy our work, if we can't stand our boss, if our work contradicts our beliefs, if our work is boring or has no meaning to us, if we aren't living our passion ... we will probably go to the fridge too often.

Optional solutions:

Work fewer hours, modify your work to the way you want it to be. Maybe you can't get rid of your boss, but maybe there are changes you can make. Resign, change your job or seriously consider the work you feel passionate about, retrain and go for it.

Relationships – If you are unhappy in your relationship, if you and your partner have grown apart, if you are staying with the wrong person for the wrong reasons, if you have unresolved issues with family members, friends, co-workers … you will probably eat way too much.

Optional solutions:

This is a tough one, especially when there are children involved. But everything is possible. First you have to look reality straight in the eye. It is always helpful to talk things over and communicate your feelings, first to yourself and then to your partner. Try to make up with the people in your life. Seek support.

Fun – Many people fall into a regular boring routine of just taking care of the kids and working.

Optional solutions:

Make your life interesting and fun! The more fun life is, the less you will eat. Make time for physical activity, reading and the activities you love. Remember how you were as a child … What did you love doing when you were young?

Whatever it is (whether it is your work, your relationships, not doing enough or the right physical activity, not having enough fun), you have to be totally honest with yourself and see what isn't working in your life. Then, recognize your fears, but bravely go for change. It is very helpful to get support to make a change in your life.

It doesn't always mean you divorce. It doesn't necessarily mean you resign from your job. You have to see what it is you can shift, modify and add. But you must decide that something has to be done!

It also might be that a very big change has to be made. And soon it might be time to LEAP.

Whatever it is, I encourage you to fully look at your life. I personally was in a life where I felt I wasn't living in a way that fulfilled me. I was compromising. Change isn't easy, but I promise you I never looked back once. I am so grateful that I had the courage and support to jump into the unknown.

Go to the Emotion

There always is a very good reason why you are turning to food or eating in an unbalanced way. Check with yourself what you are feeling, what is going on inside. If you go to the emotion, you will often find that dealing with it, feeling it, observing it and giving it space and place will release it and you won't turn to food for the wrong reasons. It is when we don't deal with what we feel that we need to fill ourselves or compensate for ourselves.

> **Remember:** There always is a very good reason why you are eating in an unbalanced way. There always is an emotion that wants to be dealt with.

Eating is always a decision. Nobody forces your hand to pick up food and put it into your mouth.

THE ART AND SCIENCE OF RATIONAL EATING

The Power Of Our Cravings/ Addictions

The addictions and cravings we have when things in our life aren't balanced (whether it's food, alcohol, smoking, shopping, physical activity – whatever it is we are addicted to in an exaggerated way) can actually help us grow and change our life for the better. If we listen to our cravings, try to understand what they are telling us and why they arise, instead of fighting and trying to control them, they can show us what it is that is out of balance. Then, if we slowly make changes in our life, these addictions will eventually vanish. They will have no need to arise.

Understanding The Untaught Language Of Our Addictions

This is a great tool I learned at IIN. If you find yourself going to X (be it food, sweets, cakes, smoking, alcohol … anything).

1. Check with yourself what it is that you are getting from X: sweetness, interest, love and affection, calmness and relaxation … it can be many different things.

2. The next step is to ask yourself, *How else can I get more of Y in my life, without going to my addiction?* For example:

   - How can I bring more sweetness into my life? (Maybe have a massage on a weekly basis.)

   - How can I make my life more interesting? (Maybe your job isn't interesting to you.)

   - How can I feel more love and affection? What is missing?

   - How can I calm and relax myself, besides going to X? (Maybe try a yoga class.)

3. Once you start bringing in Y (sweetness, interest, love and affection, calmness) on a regular basis, not only when your addiction arises, you might notice that slowly your cravings and addictions weaken and eventually vanish, since more of Y will prevent your craving from arising. The addictions and cravings will have no need to come; they only come when things are unbalanced.

Let's Go Through the Whole Process Together

This is only an example, but the structure can work for all cravings and addictions:

1. You find yourself **craving and eating many sweets**: cakes and cookies, chocolate, anything sweet.

2. Ask yourself: **What am I getting** from the sweet foods? It could be sweetness, calmness, love, or interest (for each person it will be different).

3. Ask yourself: **How else can I get more of the sweetness**, calmness, love or interest in my life, aside from going to my addiction? It could be by **adding** into my life: dancing, singing, drawing, walking in nature, meeting friends, working on a personal project ... anything that gives you the feeling of sweetness, calmness, love, interest.

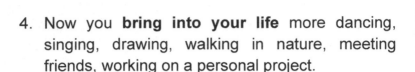

4. Now you **bring into your life** more dancing, singing, drawing, walking in nature, meeting friends, working on a personal project.

5. You might notice that after a while your cravings weaken and eventually vanish.

Step
17

This was a serious chapter. Perhaps much of what was written here, you already know. But in our lives, which are constantly growing and changing, there always is a next step that can be taken. Great questions always bring great answers. You could ask yourself one of these questions:

• What aspects of my life need to be looked at?

• Physical activity – how is that going for me? What could I do that is moving my body and fun for me?

• How is my intimate relationship? Is there

anything that could be addressed?

- Am I happy in my other relationships (with parents, kids, friends, co-workers, family)?

- What do I think about my career? Am I living my passion?

- Am I having fun? What could I do to bring more enjoyment, excitement, laughter and sweetness into my life?

- What baby step can I take this week?

When you find yourself turning to food, go to the emotion. Feel your emotions. Feel and deal with what is happening inside. You can also listen to your cravings and addictions. Even right now, before they come up – what do they give you? How could you bring more of what they give you into your life? How can you prevent them from arising in the first place?

A Few More Tips For A Powerful Life

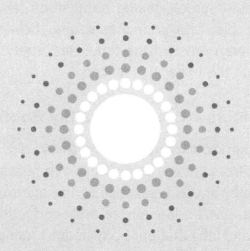

*Health is a journey,
not a destination.*

Anonymous

Though there is so much that can be written on health, here are just a few more healthy tips that I find beneficial and that you might want to use on your journey. Please take only what resonates and leave out anything that might feel too much, seem impossible or even sound boring ... and remember, don't make it into a religion. Keep things fresh and light and use your own wisdom. Continue being patient with yourself, taking baby steps, adding new healthy habits into your life, seeing how you feel. Practice them most of the time, and every now and then, break the rules. It is all fine.

Eating Hours – Create a Healthy Routine

Even though in our modern world we have disconnected ourselves from nature, like living in overheated houses in the winter and refrigerators in the summer, eating foods that aren't seasonal, or artificial foods made in factories and labs that our body doesn't recognize, our body actually works in accordance with nature. The Universe is the macro, and we are the micro. Whatever is happening outwards is also happening inwards – our bodies are constantly adjusting themselves to the outer changes and cycles. For example, between 12:00 and 13:00, the sun is highest in the sky, the hottest time of the day. At that same time of the day our digestive juices, our digestive fire (in Ayurveda, called the Agni), is also at its peak and most efficient – therefore it is the best time to eat our bigger meal (not at 22:00 at night when the body is actually in a sleeping mode). One of the important things that helps us stay balanced and energetic is to have a routine. Our body works well when there is routine. Let's talk about eating hours.

The ideal hours to eat are:

- Breakfast around 7:00-8:00

- Lunch somewhere between 12:00 noon and 13:30 (finishing at 13:30)

- Dinner between 18:00-19:00

For many people I know this seems impossible.

Earlier, we talked about breakfast being the most important meal of the day, but nothing should come between you and your lunch (the meal you could skip is dinner).

Make lunch the main meal of the day, and eat it in a relaxed manner. If you find yourself always missing, skipping and working during lunch hours, you could write it down in your diary as a lunch meeting so you don't schedule anything right before or during lunch hours. You plan it into your daily schedule: **12:30 - "EAT LUNCH."**

If you eat lunch too late, around 14:00-15:00 (and some even wait till 16:00), it is past the time when you digest best, and also you are probably already starving and eat too fast and too much. It totally throws you off balance. Instead of feeling energized, you will feel heavy, bloated and tired. It also messes up dinner, pushing it to 21:00 or 22:00 at night, and then you go to bed on a full stomach. The food isn't digested properly (since at night the body doesn't deal with digestion but rather with cleansing), and you wake up tired and still digesting last night's dinner. You aren't hungry for breakfast, and the whole cycle is messed up for the new day.

If you feel like correcting it, you could try either skipping or having a very light early dinner; you might wake up hungry for breakfast, and then schedule lunch into your day between 12:00 and 13:00.

You will notice you have much more energy and your digestive problems may slowly begin to resolve.

When I see that I do have something scheduled over my lunchtime (which seldom happens) I will usually have an early lunch, even if it is only 11:00.

Don't miss your lunch!

Sleeping Hours – Create a Healthy Routine

I used to go to sleep around midnight, sometimes even at 1:00 A.M. There were always "so many things I could do" at night. For most people that's normal. But ever since I learned that the best time to go to sleep is before 22:00, I have changed my habit. I became a morning person. I love going to sleep early and waking up early. I love the morning hours before everything begins. It is a great time to do yoga, meditate, have quiet time for myself and begin the day.

So why is it so important to go to sleep early? At night the liver cleans the blood, the time the body naturally detoxes (that is why the body isn't supposed to be digesting or even be awake for that matter). The liver and kidneys need all the energy for cleansing the blood and other important bodily functions. The most important hours for purification and renewal are between 22:00 and 24:00. If you miss out on those hours, it won't be the same sleep.

Those hours are the best for deep sleep, rest and rejuvenation. You will notice that as you slowly get used to going to sleep earlier, you will be much healthier, more energetic and more efficient in your waking hours. You will actually jump out of bed, ready to start the day.

Many people resist going to sleep and keep themselves up by eating. Many people have "a date" with the fridge when it is actually time to go to sleep. So, when you feel tired, instead of eating at night, just take yourself to bed.

Do Exercise That You Love

It is so very important to move the body. Besides making you feel good, young and fit, research shows that the health benefits may also include strengthening the bones, stimulating the growth of new brain cells, controlling blood sugar levels and aiding depression. It is also very important to find a physical activity that you really enjoy, not just doing something for the sake of exercising. Make it fun, enjoy it and then it will last, otherwise it will again be like a "diet" that you do for awhile, but isn't sustainable.

As you already know by now, baby steps are the best way to progress. Start small and what you start will eventually become a habit.

I try to move my body as much as I can. Besides taking my dog for long walks and practicing physical yoga, I also always use the stairs instead of taking the elevator, and many times I park far away so I get a chance to walk. People often go around the block five times in order to find a parking spot that is close to their destination. Why not park a bit farther away and walk? If you take the bus, get off two bus stops earlier and walk to your final destination.

Slowing Down

Modern life in the Western World is so crazy. We do so much in every day and we often stress ourselves past our limit. I want to encourage you to slow down. Schedule less. See what isn't necessary for today. Many illnesses are actually stress-related. When under stress, the body releases the stress hormone cortisol. Though cortisol in small amounts is fine and even healthy, high levels on a constant basis have many negative health-related outcomes, including decreased bone density, suppressed thyroid, elevated blood pressure, blood sugar imbalance, premature aging and even weight gain, since when the body is under stress it will not release fat and will not build muscle. Just the last two outcomes alone might make you instantly slow down.

So take deep breaths, and slow down your life. I noticed that I sometimes stressed myself by scheduling appointments too close to one other. Now, on purpose, I leave more time between them. I space them out, and so even if one is running a bit late (which often happens) I am not stressed. And I always make sure I have enough time for my lunch break.

Besides slowing down and trying to live a stress-free life as much as possible, here are a few foods which help the body adapt to stress: goji berries, maca powder, tulsi (a herb from the basil family, available as a tea) and ashwaganda (an Ayurvedic Indian herb).

Food For Thought: We work stressfully all our life to gain wealth and then we use all our wealth to try and gain back our health.

TV and Newspapers

Watching TV and reading the daily newspaper can be quite toxic and stressful for the body and mind, though when we're absorbed in the activity, we aren't aware of it. Today I barely watch TV and never buy a paper. When you free yourself from being addicted to the news first thing in the morning or being a couch potato at night, you find there are many other things you can do that really fulfill and nourish you (which can also include going to sleep earlier).

I want to strongly remind you not to eat in front of the TV. A research study conducted with kids found that while they were watching TV and had food put in front of them, they were so absorbed they ate things that they normally weren't willing to touch: vegetables. In this case, the unaware eating just happened to be healthy! (So if your kids do watch TV and you would like to get them eating more vegetables, maybe in this case you can take advantage of the lack of awareness and put out a plate of cut cucumbers and carrots).

It is also better to find the exact program you want to watch rather than just zap between different channels and suddenly realize the whole evening went by. You can also tape an interesting show to watch later.

Here Comes the Sun

> *The fact that an opinion has been widely held is no evidence whatever that it is not utterly absurd.*
>
> Bertrand Russell

There was a time I used to be terrified of the sun. I would avoid going out during mid-day and when I did I would wear long clothes and a big hat, put tons of sunscreen on my face and body and walk in the shady areas. For some time now I have felt liberated, ever since I "became sober" and learned not only that the sun is essential and actually very healthy but also that the thing you want to avoid using is sunscreen, full of toxic chemicals, preventing the body from creating Vitamin D.

In the summer I still wear my hat but no sunscreen, enjoying nature's healing power – the heat of the sun – letting my body soak it in and generating Vitamin D, produced when UVB sunlight hits the cholesterol in the skin. Vitamin D is crucial for calcium absorption, for preventing osteoporosis, depression and different cancers, for strengthening the immune system and so much more! And it is free.

Yet even in hot sunny countries, most people today are deficient in Vitamin D and have to take supplements. This isn't surprising since we go from our house to the car, from the car to the office, from the office back to the car (the rays of the sun which generate Vitamin D production do not penetrate glass), and when we are outdoors we put on sunscreen.

Different studies show that there is no connection between sun exposure and skin cancer and other related diseases; on the contrary, people who lack sunshine have more cancer than those who are often exposed to the sun and who live in high UVB radiation areas near the equator. Actually, UVB radiation can prevent cancer.*

Therefore, I recommend getting a balanced dose of sunshine. The best hours for UVB radiation are at mid-day (20-40 minutes a day, depending on the time of the year – in winter even more) and depending on your skin color (the darker you are, the longer you have to be in the sun). You don't want to burn your skin, but getting it a bit pinkish, gradually toning to a darker color, is very healthy. For more information on

---

Timeless Secrets of Health & Rejuvenation by Andreas Moritz, Chapter 8 "Healing Secrets of the Sun."

this subject please refer to one of the books I most personally value: *Timeless Secrets of Health and Rejuvenation* by Andreas Moritz.

Grounding

I am told that when I was small I always wanted to walk around barefoot. I would take off my shoes whenever I could, and my parents would try to get me to put them back on. I was thought to be headstrong. Today, I realize I actually had very good instincts and it was my parents who should have been taking off their shoes.

Do you know what one of humanity's worst innovations is? Funnily enough, it's rubber-soled shoes. The Earth has an electromagnetic field that is very important for our health and well being, but we actually are barely connected to it anymore. We all walk on rubber soles (you hardly find shoes with leather soles anymore), have carpets and floor tiles in the house, drive in cars and so on.

When was the last time you walked barefoot on the planet? There is something so natural and healing about walking barefoot – being in contact with and feeling the earth beneath, absorbing the natural vibrations, energy and electricity of the planet. The effect upon us is that it discharges electrical stress that we accumulate and it restores the body's natural and stable electrical state. Being aware of this, you actually can feel yourself feeling better. Grounding our body is beneficial in dealing with chronic pain, back problems, cancer, inflammation and more. Even while talking on a cellular phone or working at the computer, it is beneficial to be grounded, being barefoot and connected to the earth.

How to ground yourself naturally:

- Take your shoes off.

- Walk barefoot on the beach, sand, earth or grass for at least 30 minutes at a time. Even if you live in the city, find a bench in a park, take off your shoes and feel the earth beneath you.

- Go into the sea, a river or lake (connecting to natural water is one of the most grounding things you can do).

- Eat root vegetables or vegetables which grow at ground level: pumpkins, sweet potatoes, beets, carrots, onions, ginger.

- Gardening – work in your garden or at a friend's garden. They will appreciate it, and so will your body. Grow herbs and plants on your balcony, getting your fingers into the earth.

- Practice yoga. People who begin practicing yoga on a regular basis report a sense of grounding in their body and their emotions. Feeling stronger, healthier, with more energy, having greater focus.

Have a routine that is healthy and fun for you – try to go to sleep and wake up at the same hours, eat at the same times, exercise regularly and do any other practice that makes you feel good, whether it is yoga, meditation, dancing, painting – you will notice a big difference in your health and happiness.

Food for Thought: When I go walking with my dog, Dova, she always pulls to walk on the earth. She doesn't like walking on the cement or sidewalks. I wonder: Does Dova have the instinct to ground herself – one that we once had but have lost?

Healthy Toothpaste

I was shocked to find out what unhealthy ingredients are in regular toothpastes. Isn't it the weirdest thing in the world that all regular toothpastes have a similar warning on them: *"Do Not Swallow. Children under six years of age should use only a pea-size amount and be supervised while brushing"*?

Doesn't that raise some questions? Is this toothpaste or poison? Many regular toothpastes have a long list of harmful, toxic, carcinogenic ingredients in them. To name just a few:

- Triclosan – a pesticide.

- Sodium Laurel Sulfate, SLS – it is what produces the bubbles and foam. But it is also used in garages and car washes for melting and cleaning off grease!

- Fluoride, colorants (blues, greens and reds made from tar) and even different kinds of sweeteners: saccharin, sorbitol (sometimes it is even the first ingredient on the list).**

I highly recommend switching to a natural healthy toothpaste that doesn't taste sweet (has no sugar in it) and doesn't foam. There are natural salt toothpastes on the market (after a while you get used to and like them) or others made from plants (even though the label claims it is "natural," always read the ingredient list). Salt- and plant-based toothpaste is also very

---

** *The Oral Health Bible* by Michael P.Bonner (D.D.S) & Earl L. Mindell (R.Ph., Ph.D).

beneficial for healthy gums and discourages the growth of oral bacteria. After just a short period of use, you will notice the change. Once you switch to a more natural toothpaste and then go back to regular toothpaste, it actually feels like you are brushing your teeth in sugar and your whole mouth is one big bubble of chemicals.

The Tongue Cleaner

A great and simple tool from the Indian Ayurveda tradition is the tongue cleaner. It is a metal hand-held U-shaped tool that you scrape over your tongue to clean it. I find it is life-transforming. I have been using it for years, ever since I went to India in my early 20s, and now I wouldn't brush my teeth without it. During the night many toxins are released, and many of them accumulate on the tongue. Before brushing your teeth in the morning, scrape off the toxins, plaque and build-up using the tongue cleaner. I don't recommend using the toothbrush to brush your tongue; it doesn't do the job. The tongue cleaner may be purchased at some pharmacies and yoga stores.

Step
18

We are at Step 18 – Congratulations!

So ... what is your next step?

Creating a routine? Adjusting your eating hours or sleeping hours? Finding and doing exercise that you enjoy? How can you de-stress and slow down? Could you cut out some TV hours? How are you doing with the newspaper? Can you be more in the sun? Are you using sunscreen? Are you grounding yourself? What toothpaste are you using? Will you buy a tongue cleaner?

Yoga Saved My Life!

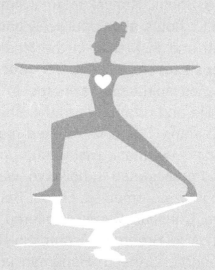

The tragedy of the soul is that it would rather fail in someone else's story than succeed in its own.

Anonymous

Between the ages of 20 and 34 I was in India at least ten times. I was in Pune at OSHO's ashram many times, changed my name and took all kinds of different courses and experienced dynamic meditations. I traveled from the northernmost part of India, from Leh, down to the point where "the land ends" in the South, Kanyakumari. I smoked ganja and danced for hours at colorful lively parties, in Goa in the South and in Manali in the North. I trekked in the (Nepalese) mountains for weeks. I read many books on spirituality, awareness, inner work, meditation, life and death. I read the Bhagavad Gita and learned some Sanskrit. I visited many spiritual cities (including Varanasi, Rishikesh, Jaislamer and Udaipur) and participated in holidays, weddings and different religious ceremonies: Hindu, Buddhist, Jain, Sikh, Muslim, Christian, Jewish. I offered flowers and other offerings to Brahma, Vishnu, Shiva, Lakshmi, Krishna, Buddha, Ganesh, Hanuman and others. I visited castles, monasteries, churches, ashrams and one synagogue. I sang, drummed and chanted in different singing circles, learned reiki, made chapatti, chanted the OM, put my hands in Namaste ... But somehow, I didn't go to even ONE yoga class.

It was only back in Tel Aviv, at the age of 34, when I felt that my life was going down the wrong path, that on one Saturday afternoon I found myself at a yoga class on Ben-Gurion Boulevard, in a yoga center that was a five-minute walk from my small, noisy, expensive rented apartment. Life changed instantly.

I left the class feeling like a grey cloud had lifted from above my head. I felt very light, full of trust in life and happy for no reason whatsoever. Nine years have gone by, and the cloud has never come back. Over the years my yoga practice has grown and become an innate part of me and my life.

So many people worldwide are attracted to practicing yoga; there are centers everywhere and many different yoga styles. I feel the reason for the increase in interest in yoga is that we have gone so far away from ourselves and from what truly nourishes and nurtures us that more and more souls are searching for meaning. When I say yoga, I mean much more than just the yoga poses. Yoga isn't just an acrobatic exercise. It can totally transform your life and connect you back to YOU.

Yoga is a physical way of doing spiritual work. Through breathing and accessing different areas of the body, lengthening and relaxing our physical structure, deep emotional, subconscious changes occur. It is like having an inner shower. I don't think I know of one person practicing yoga who hasn't been transformed, becoming calmer, more centered and happier.

After a year of practicing yoga daily, I decided to take a yoga teacher's training course. Not necessarily to become a teacher but to deepen both my understanding of the philosophy and my own yoga practice. I found my teacher, Shimon Ben Avi, very soon after. Over the years I learned the deep meaning of yoga. I feel grateful to the yoga philosophy and way of life for helping me make the change and take the big leap into the unknown. In the manner of the quote at the beginning of this chapter, which Shimon often mentions in his classes and is taken from different spiritual philosophies, I had been failing in someone else's story (acting, movies) instead of succeeding in my own story.

It is difficult for me to put into words the benefits of practicing yoga. Here are just two principles from amongst many others (which aren't taught in Western culture) that have become a part of me through the journey of yoga, awareness and meditation.

Abhyasa-Vairagya (Effort Versus Relaxation)

This means to make an effort but at the same time to let go, to relax. Effort (Abhyasa), but relax (Vairagya) from within. Do the yoga poses without effort, while letting go. When I had just begun practicing yoga,

I was tremendously inflexible. I often suffered from lower back pains. During the first few years I really wanted to become flexible (I would notice all the flexible girls practicing near me), and I sometimes pushed my body into certain poses. As you deepen into the yoga practice, you understand that that is contrary to the yoga way.

Yoga is observing the body as it is, without pushing it into a certain pose. Without wanting anything specific. Letting the body slowly relax into the Asana (pose). And wherever your body is now is exactly right. Understanding and practicing that on your mat will bring that same essence into your life too, quite the opposite concept to how we live in the West where it is all about effort, effort, effort. Go, go, go!! Yoga is learning how to live without effort - still "doing" (Abhyasa) while "letting go" (Vairagya) from within. Letting go of what you want the result to be. Letting life show you the way. Letting what has to happen manifest on its own. Just putting yourself in the asana, and breathing. You are exactly where you need to be. The rest will happen. It is so much nicer, calmer and relaxing to live life that way. We should be taught that in primary school.

Breathe!

Today people don't breathe, not deeply. Our breath is very shallow and becomes more and more shallow as we age. If we start noticing our breath, we will see that it is actually a bridge between the conscious and the subconscious. When we are happy and relaxed, our breath is deeper and calm; when we are nervous or angry, we will breathe more quickly and shallowly; if we are scared, we will hold our breath.

Our breath is a wonderful tool to work with, both on the yoga mat and in our life. In yoga we breathe deeply. We lengthen and observe our breath.

 Try this gentle yoga exercise:

Sit comfortably. Lengthen your spine. Slightly pull your stomach in and up. Feel the center of your body. Feel your breath going up, from the bottom of your pelvis up to the tip of your head. Follow your breath going back down. Hold your breath but stay aware and calm. Start breathing again.

Practicing breathing on the mat will help you bring your awareness back to your breath in daily life. Notice that when you breathe, "you" are doing nothing – the body is breathing on its own. If at anytime in your daily life, you find yourself stressed, thinking too much or worried, just bring your attention back to your breath, to your nostrils and to the area below the nostrils. Feel the air going in and out, in and out, and notice how you slowly calm down.

Step
19

Find some kind of practice, whether it is yoga, meditation, Tai Chi, Chi Kong, dancing, drawing, singing, walking on the beach, walking in nature, bike riding – anything at all that connects you to you, to your breath, that takes you beyond the physical world of "doing and achieving and being someone and getting somewhere," to just "being." And practice it daily. Start with a few minutes a day or every few days and gradually let it grow.

As my teacher, Joshua Rosenthal, always says, *"We are spiritual beings in a material world."*

So, spiritual being, what will it be? What is your next step in the material world?

The Last Course

The more you praise and celebrate your life,
the more there is in life to celebrate.

Oprah Winfrey

Well, we have arrived at our Last Course. But remember: Every last course will at some time have a first course that will follow later. At any time, you can start again or refer back to certain chapters.

We started our journey together quite a while ago. So much has happened, and you are doing an amazing job. How do I know? I know! This applies even if you read the book in one go. Please take a moment and remember where you were, how you felt when we began and where you are today.

Please Take a Moment …

It is so very important to acknowledge our achievements along the way, even if in our mind we have that voice that says "you didn't achieve anything". If you still have those strong voices, please refer back to Step 3 "Staying In The Positive Zone" on page 33.

Here is your last step for now. This is a table to help you acknowledge where you are and what you have achieved so far. Please fill in the column on the right:

Step No.	The Baby Step to Take	The Baby Steps I Took and Where I Am Today
1	Read the first chapter in "Have a Superlife"	
2	Sign contract: I commit that I will pay close attention to what I say and what I commit to; I will do my best to stand up to my word.	
3	Keep myself in a positive half-full cup mode	Am I more positive? What do I use?
4	Some basic health information: microwaving/stove, plastic containers/glass, sugar and artificial sweeteners, sodas and diet drinks/water, processed foods/whole foods, oils, salt, reading labels, organic produce, products from the animal kingdom, cleaning products	What info did I incorporate?
5	Food equipment list: large salad bowl, small bowl, smoothie glass, blender, pressure cooker	Which of these did I incorporate into my kitchen. What did I get? What am I using?

Step No.	The Baby Step to Take	The Baby Steps I Took and Where I Am Today
6	Ingredient list: greens, sprouts, vegetables, sweet vegetables, whole grains, fruits, dried fruits, nuts, legumes, spices, seeds, oils, seaweeds, tahini, superfoods, healthy sweeteners	What ingredients did I add? How am I eating differently?
7	Upgrade your food – superfoods	Which superfoods do I use?
8	Breakfast	Am I eating breakfast? What has changed?
9	Basic summer meal	Have I changed my lunch? Am I eating big salads? Greens?
10	Basic winter meal	Did I make the Super Soup/Stew?
11	Cooking	Do I cook more? What am I cooking?

Step No.	The Baby Step to Take	The Baby Steps I Took and Where I Am Today
12	Healthy snacks	Have I changed my snacks?
13	How to eat	Am I chewing? Am I eating with more awareness?
14	Healthy on the go	Am I making healthy choices when eating out? Am I taking food to work? Do I make a lunchbox?
15	Whole grains	Which whole grains am I eating? Do I eat less processed grains?
16	Legumes and sprouting	Which legumes am I eating? Do I sprout?

Step No.	The Baby Step to Take	The Baby Steps I Took and Where I Am Today
17	Making my life healthy – not only my food	What changes did I make in the different aspects of my life?
18	Healthy living tips	What did I incorporate?
19	My practice	What practice have I incorporated into my life? What do I do that connects me more to me? Do I observe my breath?
20		Overall, what other changes have I taken? What do I appreciate myself for? How will I celebrate finishing the book?

Look At All You Have Accomplished!!!! BRAVO to You!!

Please remember:

This Is a Lifelong Journey

Focus on making this sustainable, a lifelong way of eating and living. Even if you haven't achieved everything you set out to achieve, focus on what you have accomplished; recognize, congratulate and acknowledge yourself for what you have obtained and what you are doing.

Be Patient With Yourself

Remember that you learned a new language and like any new thing, it takes practice, persistence and patience.

Progress - Not Perfection

Focus on your progress, don't try to perfect life. Focusing on the progress keeps it light and fun and keeps you happy; focusing on perfection makes it heavy and rigid and makes you seriously unhappy. Don't sell your happiness away for anything!

Slow Down

Allow the change to be gradual. Once you feel comfortable with your new habit, bring in another one. Reread this book as many times as you need, creating new healthy habits each time.

Baby, Baby, Baby Steps

Break your steps down to enjoyable baby ones – but still, you must take those steps. Then celebrate each little step you achieved. How will you celebrate today?

Simplify Things

Choose the simple path, the one of least resistance. Try to make it simple. Usually there is an easy path we can choose. Always ask yourself, How can I simplify this? How can I break it down into even smaller steps? How can I make it easy and fun for me?

Listen to Life – It Will Show You the Way

If something you want isn't happening, and you have tried to get it many times – then maybe it is time to let it go! Many people won't agree with me, since we live in a society that says things like, "Don't give up," "Work hard," "No one said life is easy". But from my personal experience – when I was in my early 30s and I tried to achieve all kinds of different things over and over and over again and they weren't happening and the process wasn't giving me any pleasure – it is only when I let it go that something else even better took its place. It doesn't necessarily mean to let go of it totally; it can mean, "let it go for now," "take a break," "try to achieve it from a different place."

It isn't letting go of what you **want**, it is letting go of **the way you think it should happen** and opening yourself to other possibilities that you might be missing out on, when you are so determined to get what it is, the way you want it. This occurred in so many different aspects of my life, and still does today. When something isn't happening, I stop. It is a sign from life, and I see what is actually being presented to me. Life always shows the way.

> That is why I say "Listen To Life". It will show you the way. Choose the easy path.

Easy doesn't mean that you don't have to work, but it means that as you put in your energy, your time, your work … things seem to flow. The doors are opening for you. You are not knocking and finding no-one. That is how I simplify things. I put a lot of energy into what

I do, but I let go of the things that aren't happening. This isn't always easy to do. Then the right thing or the right way of achieving my intention comes along, so I take it. And it is easy. And it is simple. See life as it is, not as you would like it to be.

Try Not to Identify So Much

It helps to remind ourselves that we aren't our cars, houses, clothes, jobs – we aren't even our own body. It helps to look at things a bit from a distance.

You Are the Focus

Put the focus on yourself, on what you feel is good and right for you. Listen to your feelings, your body – your personal lab. Only **YOU** know best what is right for you. Being somewhat egoistical is actually a healthy thing. You care about others, but you still do what is right and healthy for you.

It Doesn't Have to Be 100% Healthy

Go for a 20 percent – 80 percent diet.

Try a 70 to 80 percent healthy one (of homemade food, fruits, vegetables, whole grains, legumes, superfoods) and a 20 to 30 percent diet of what you know isn't totally healthy but is what you LOVE.

Much more fun. Far more sustainable. Very important!

Thank You

I want to thank you for giving me the opportunity to share my personal life experiences and support you on your path towards health and happiness.

You are doing a great job. I am here for you whenever you want to start again, read a certain chapter or to just have a little reminder. I recommend to always keep on adding new healthy habits, one step at a time. I myself do that all the time.

You are also welcome to join the "have a Superl!fe" mailing list.

Now it is time **TO CELEBRATE!**

Together we can all have a Superl!fe.

With health, love and inspiration,

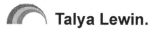 **Talya Lewin.**

A Few More Of My Favorite Recipes

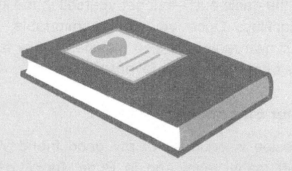

Changing our diet is more powerful than what we imagine.

Neal Barnard

As you know by now, though I love eating, I don't spend much time in the kitchen. I don't cook gourmet. On a daily basis I cook very simple, tasty and healthy meals. Most of my daily dishes are included throughout the book, but here are a few more. They all are REALLY easy, so just pick up the ingredients, stand in the kitchen, turn on some music and have fun.

Even if you are missing one or two ingredients … DO NOT LET THAT STOP YOU! Use something else or "leave the garlic out" – but get yourself in the kitchen and cooking. Once you feel comfortable, make up your own recipes. I also included a few favorite recipes from some of my favorite people.

Another Smoothie

This recipe is courtesy of my good friend Vishva. We met many years ago in Pune, India. He now lives in Portugal, spending his time researching health and nutrition. If you ever have any serious illness, Vishva would be the person to contact: **vishvaji@yahoo.com**.

This is a great light summer lunch or dinner option.

Savory Green Smoothie

Ingredients – for 1 serving:

- 2 very ripe juicy tomatoes – most important

- 1 cucumber

- 1/2 zucchini

- A bunch of parsley, a bit of coriander, arugula

- 1/4 onion

- 1 small garlic clove

- 1 tsp. flax seeds or 1 tsp. chia seeds

- 1 Tbsp. pine nuts

- 1 Tbsp. soaked and peeled almonds – optional

- 1 Tbsp. coconut oil

- 1 Tbsp. olive oil

- Himalayan salt

- 2-3 ice cubes

- You can also add spirulina, kelp, chlorella

Directions:

1. Put chia or flax seeds in blender with a bit of water to soak.

2. Add all ingredients except the ice.

3. Start to blend, turn on high to become smooth.

4. Add ice and blend till it is very smooth.

5. Pour into a tall glass or cup and drink/eat with a long spoon.

Salads, of course

I love this cooling salad in the summer. It is so quick and easy! Always keep a cooked grain in the fridge, and in minutes you will make yourself a delicious nutritious meal.

No need to stick to the recipe – you can play around with the vegetables you have in the fridge. It also works great with other grains like brown rice, millet and kasha.

Green Speedy Quinoa Salad

Ingredients - for 3 servings:

- 2 cups cooked quinoa (try mixing the red and white varieties)

- 1/2 cup chopped red pepper

- 1/2 cup chopped cucumber

- 1/2 cup chopped fresh dill (leaves and stems)

- 1/2 cup chopped celery (leaves and stalks)

- 1/2 cup chopped fresh mint (leaves)

- 1/2 cup chopped fresh parsley (leaves and stems)

- 1/2 cup chopped fresh coriander (leaves and stems)

- Any leafy greens you love or have in the fridge

Dressing:

No amounts! Just follow your instinct till it tastes right:

- Olive oil

- Lemon juice

- Himalayan salt

- Freshly ground black pepper

- Ground cumin

Directions:

Combine all ingredients together in a large bowl and mix well.

Another Great Simple Salad

Ingredients - for 1 serving:

- 1/4 purple cabbage, sliced thin (it is so beautiful in the salad)

- 1 green onion, bunch of mint leaves – chopped

- 1 carrot – peeled lengthwise into long strips (looks amazing with the purple)

- Mung bean sprouts (or any other bean sprouts)

Dressing: (the trick is in the dressing, making it thick and coating everything)

- Juice of 1 lemon

- 1-2 Tbsp. tahini

- 1 tsp. olive oil

- 1 tsp. sesame oil

- 1-2 Tbsp. soy sauce

Directions:

1. Put all the veggies in a big bowl.

2. Pour the dressing straight onto the salad.

3. Mix well.

4. You might have to add more of some of the dressing ingredients.

5. Eat with awareness, using chopsticks.

Remember to always rotate the veggies you eat.

Spreads

I don't think a day goes by for me without eating tahini. Here is an unusual and delicious recipe for tahini made from whole sesame seeds (not hulled, of course), which is a great source of calcium and protein. It can be used as a spread or as a salad dressing, if liquefied.

Sweet Tahini

Ingredients - for 5 servings:

- 1/2 cup whole sesame tahini

- 1/2 cup mandarin juice (you can chop and add the remaining fruit pulp)

- Bunch of dill – leaves and stems, chopped

Directions:

1. In a bowl, hand mix together the tahini and mandarin juice until well combined.

2. It will look separated at first: just keep whisking!

3. Add the chopped dill and mix.

4. Add additional juice or some water if you want a thinner consistency.

5. Serve over grains, bread, cooked vegetables, greens or salad.

Note: Keeps refrigerated for about five days.

Lettuce Leaf Sandwich – The Bread Is Only the Filling

This is one of my mother's inventions. I saw her eating it for some time and never thought much of it. But once I tried it, I realized it is ingenious! You can make it with any filling of your choice. Here is the basic idea:

Ingredients – for 1 serving:

- 1 very large Romaine lettuce leaf, from the outer leaves

- 1 slice whole grain bread, lightly toasted

- Avocado slices

- Tomato slices or roasted red pepper

- Arugula, sprouts, or chopped fresh coriander

- Chopped green onion

- Flavorings: lemon juice, freshly ground black pepper, Himalayan salt, etc.

Directions:

1. Place the slice of bread on the lettuce leaf, 3/4 of the way down.

2. Layer with the vegetable filling of your choice.

3. Drizzle with a bit of lemon juice, and add flavorings.

4. Fold up the bottom and sides of the lettuce leaf to envelop the bread and filling, and hold tightly.

Note: It is a bit messy, and once you start eating you can't put it down. But it's a great way to have a delicious sandwich with only one piece of bread.

Remember to chew and eat slowly.

Other Dishes to Put on Top of the Salad

Stewed Rice-Filled Red Peppers

Ingredients – for 6 servings:

- 6 medium red peppers
- 1 cup whole brown rice –soak overnight, rinse and drain
- 1 tomato
- 1 onion
- 2-3 cloves garlic
- A lot of parsley
- A lot of coriander
- 2 tsp. cumin
- 1 tsp. turmeric
- 1/8 tsp. cayenne
- 1/2 tsp. salt
- Freshly ground black pepper
- 2 Tbsp. tomato paste

»

- 2 Tbsp. olive oil

Sauce

Ingredients:

- 2 Tbsp. olive oil

- 1 onion

- 1 tomato

- 3 Tbsp. tomato paste

- 1 tsp. cumin

- 1 1/2 cup water

Directions:

1. Soak rice overnight, rinse and drain.

2. Cut tops off peppers and remove seeds.

3. Chop onion, tomato, garlic, parsley, coriander, plus flesh from pepper tops; add to rice with cumin, turmeric, cayenne, salt, pepper, tomato paste and olive oil and mix well.

4. Fill peppers with rice mixture.

5. In saucepan, sauté chopped onion in olive oil, add chopped tomato, tomato paste, spice and water to make a sauce. Add any remaining rice mixture.

6. Place peppers in sauce, cover and simmer about one hour and fifteen minutes, turning a few times, adding water as needed. Check that rice is tender.

7. Serve with freshly chopped coriander.

Soups

This is my mother's cook-in-the-soup's-own-heat method. It is very quick and a healthy way to keep all vegetables nutritious and colorful.

Presto-Steamed Vegetable Soup - Basic Recipe

Ingredients:

- Olive oil

- Onions

- Carrots

- Zucchini

- Various additions, of your choice:
  potatoes, yams, leeks + tops, peas, turnips
  (peeled), peppers, garlic, jalapeno pepper,
  tomatoes, pumpkin, squash

- Bunch of chopped parsley and/or dill,
  including stems

- Boiling water to cover (can add saved
  water from previously steamed vegetables
  - too nutritious to discard!)

- Flavorings: soy sauce, fresh ginger,
  cayenne, sea salt, pepper, cumin, other
  fresh herbs like coriander, oregano – your
  choice

»

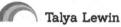

- Optional: cooked beans, lentils

Directions:

1. Cut unpeeled vegetables into small to medium-sized pieces.

2. Sauté onion in olive oil, add carrots, potatoes, and other longer cooking vegetables.

3. Add boiling water and any other vegetables and bring to a boil.

4. Cover pot and turn off heat – you will be surprised that it "cooks" quite quickly.

5. Remove cover when vegetables are just softened and the colors are still bright.

6. Add freshly chopped parsley and/or dill and other fresh herbs and mix well.

7. If desired, blend while hot with handheld blender, until as smooth as you want it.

8. To the basic recipe, add any combination of flavorings desired.

9. Cooked beans or lentils may also be added (before or after blending).

Desserts & Snacks

While growing up my mother always baked delicious cakes and especially apple cakes. Later on I opened my cake business based on her apple cake. But as my diet changed and became healthier, my close family became influenced too. My mother started cooking and baking healthier recipes. Here are two of her delicious apple recipes:

Stove-Top Stewed Apples

Ingredients – for 6 servings:

- 6 stewing apples
- 1-2 oranges (zest of 1, juice and chopped pulp of 2)
- 1/4 cup dried cranberries (unsweetened)
- 1 tsp. cinnamon

Directions:

1. Without peeling, core and cut the apples into big chunks and put in a cooking pot.
2. Add all ingredients and combine well.

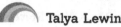

3. Cook covered, starting on a low heat, careful not to burn.

4. As juices begin to flow, turn up heat and when it starts to boil, turn heat off and leave covered – it will cook in its own heat.

5. Remove lid when apples are softened.

This dish remains chunky and still has the nutritious edible apple skins.

This can also be oven-baked for some additional caramelized flavor.

Enjoy warm or as a very cold dessert.

Oven-Baked Apples

Ingredients – for 6 servings:

- 6 baking apples
- 2 oranges (zest of 1 orange, juice and chopped pulp of 2 oranges)
- 1/3 cup dried cranberries
- 1/3 cup pistachios
- 1 tsp. cinnamon

Directions:

1. Without peeling, core apples and place in a Pyrex baking dish.

2. Mix cranberries, pistachios, zest and chopped pulp and fill the hollows.

3. Mix cinnamon with orange juice and pour over each apple, adding the remainder to the dish.

4. Bake at 200C/350F for approximately 45 minutes until apples soften.

>>

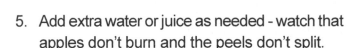
5. Add extra water or juice as needed - watch that apples don't burn and the peels don't split.

Enjoy warm or as a very cold dessert.

The Best Banana Ice Cream – All Natural!

Ingredients - for 2 servings:

- 2 ripe bananas – peel, cut and freeze
- Topping of your choice

Directions:

1. Blend frozen bananas in food processor or blender until very creamy, push the fruit well into the blade and blend some more.

2. Transfer to two bowls, and sprinkle with the topping of your choice: cacao nibs, goji berries, mulberries, nuts, raisins, a shake of cinnamon, whole sesame tahini paste, maple syrup, silan … you can't go wrong.

Enjoy the tastiest, healthiest ice cream on the planet!

My Favorite Finter (Fall + Winter) Snack

This tastes like cake, actually even better.

Ingredients - for 2 servings:

- 2 sweet potatoes
- Sauce: homemade tahini or olive oil with soy sauce (additional cinnamon is optional).

Directions:

1. Cut the sweet potatoes into thick, 2-3 cm slices.

2. Using a vegetable steamer basket, steam for 5-7 minutes or until soft, paying attention not to overcook.

3. Move to a plate and spread each slice with Homemade Tahini Sauce, or drizzle with olive oil and soy sauce.

4. For an extra blood sugar stabilizer you can add a bit of cinnamon.

Who needs processed cakes and cookies and hydrogenated oils when you can have this? It is the best snack ever!

Step
21

Did you find any recipe that inspired you to get into the kitchen again? Or maybe to invent a dish of you own? Do you know anyone else reading this book? You could each make one of the recipes and then share them.

Have fun and keep in touch!

THANK YOU!

My close family was really involved in getting this book out. I want to thank you all:

Cynie – My super super mother, who is always there for me, no matter what. Thank you for everything you did, do and will do for me in this lifetime, and also for supporting me the whole way through writing this book, going over my first to tenth (at least) draft, editing them over and over and over again, always staying loyal to my voice but adding your great tips and ideas.

Jacques – My one and only father, who left us way too soon. You had such a major role in my childhood and my overall attitude towards life. You were so easy going, so much fun, full of stories, always joking, you had so much happiness. I am so lucky to have had you as a father. Abba – I wish you were here to celebrate life with us and much more.

Diarmuid - My wonderful, supportive and loving partner for life, my husband, whom I met while writing this book. I feel so lucky that we met, and though we are from such different backgrounds, cultures, countries and climates, took the chance to be together. Life is so much fun together! Thank you for being exactly as you are. Thank you for all your help and support.

298

Oraya - Sadie – Our beautiful daughter who came to the world just as the book was being first published in Israel, and brought so much light and happiness to us all. Thank you for coming to us.

Nomi – My most amazing, wonderful, creative sister, who has always been there for me, since we were young, with intelligent and calming advice. Thank you for reading the English version, then the Hebrew one, giving your great suggestions and ideas. Thank you for helping and supporting me through so many different things in life.

Bobbie - Sadie – My wonderful special, centered, inspiring grandmother. You were and will always be an inspiration. Both in the way you lived and in the way you died. We will always miss you.

Other special people who made this book possible:

Joshua Rosenthal – My great mentor. You really made it happen. Going to IIN and having your great influence, teachings, way of thinking and support has affected a central part of this book and of me becoming who I am. Thank you for your brilliant input, ideas and tips, and for agreeing right away to write the foreword. I deeply appreciate everything.

List of Recommended Books

There are so many great books on the subject of health and nutrition.

Here are a few of my favorites:

Diabetes - No More!, Andreas Moritz

Eat Fat Lose Fat, Mary Enig and Sally Fallon

Eat to Live, Joel Fuhrman

Green for Life, Victoria Boutenko

Fast Food Nation, Eric Schlosser

Food and Healing, Annemarie Colbin

Food Rules, Michael Pollan

Healing With Wholefoods, Paul Pitchford

In Defense of Food, Michael Pollen

Integrative Nutrition, Joshua Rosenthal

Naked Chocolate, David Wolfe and Shazzie

Take Control of Your Health, Elaine Hollingsworth

The China Study, Thomas Campbell and T. Colin Campbell

The Feel Good Factor, Patrick Holford

The Omnivore's Dilemma, Michael Pollan

The Sunfood Diet Success System, David Wolfe

The Self Healing Cookbook, Kristina Turner

The Slow Down Diet, Marc David

Timeless Secrets of Health and Rejuvenation, Andreas Moritz

What to Eat, Marion Nestle

CPSIA information can be obtained at www.ICGtesting.com
Printed in the USA
BVOW11s1118110915

417593BV00025B/342/P